PRIMAL PANCREAS

Pancreas Damage Survival Guide

A. Toxopeus

Primal Pancreas
Pancreas Damage Survival Guide

ISBN: 978-0-9600679-1-6 Paperback
ISBN: 978-0-9600679-0-9 Ebook

Library of Congress Control Number: 2018968618
Published in the United States of America

DISCLAIMER: The information, subjects, ideas, concepts and opinions expressed in this book are intended to be used for educational purposes only. This is not a medical manual. If you suspect that you have a medical issue, seek professional medical help. The author and publisher are not rendering medical advice or professional services of any kind. This book is not intended to replace medical advice, nor to diagnose, prescribe, or treat any injury, disease, condition, or illness. Any sample diagnostic test results are for illustration only and cannot be used for any other purposes, including litigation. It is vital that before beginning any health, supplementation, exercise, diet or lifestyle program, including any aspect of the thoughts, ideas, opinions and recommendations mentioned in this book, you receive full medical clearance from a licensed and qualified medical professional. The author and publisher claim no responsibility to any person or entity for any liability, inferences drawn, loss or damage caused or alleged to be caused directly or indirectly as a result of the use, application or interpretation of any of the material in this book.

The author and publisher have not received any incentives, endorsements or monetary benefit from any of the books, articles, websites, studies, laboratories, items, supplements, medicines, doctors, organizations or companies mentioned in this book. Information offered was believed to be accurate at the time of publication, and neither the author nor the publisher can accept any legal responsibility, loss, damage, disruption or liability for any errors or omissions.

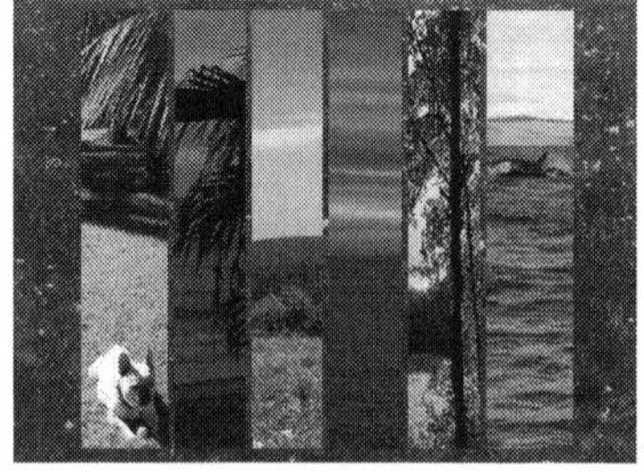

www.PrimalPancreas.com

Table of Contents

This book would not have been possible without Amy, my angel of a wife, who stuck with me and helped keep me alive through all these tough years!

Introduction

Any chronic fatigue, pain, inflammation or malaise?	Difficulty figuring out why you feel so unwell?
Any unexplained numbness, heart rhythm, paresthesia, neurotransmitter, anxiety, or breathing type issues?	Any premature aging issues such as bone density, low hormones, low energy, or difficulty healing issues?
Any intestinal issues like malabsorption, bloating, irritable bowel, bacterial or yeast overgrowth?	Any unexplained nutrient deficiencies, microbiome dysbiosis, reflux, or food sensitivities like gluten?
Any pancreas damage issues such as atrophy, pancreatitis, diabetes, or exocrine pancreatic insufficiency?	Not getting clear answers for unexplained or chronic symptoms, even after many tests and dead ends?
Interested in potential causes of modern chronic ailments?	Interested in practical steps to help your body heal?

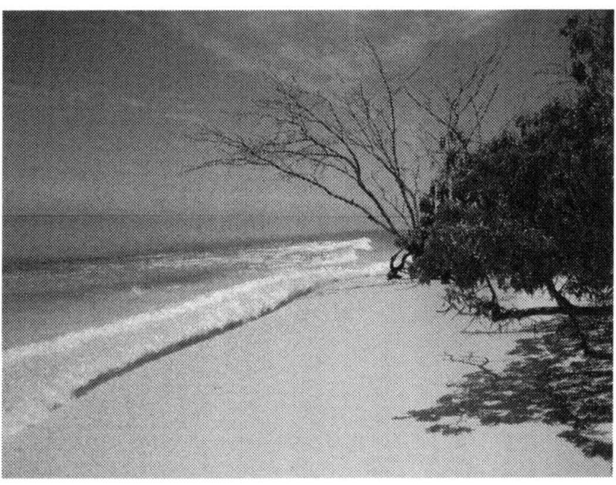

If you answered yes to any of these questions, please continue reading. This book is meant as a practical guide and as a source of reference information for doctors and sufferers of pancreatic damage and malabsorption. Many ailments, from which millions are suffering, including the ones in the questions above, are often not linked to the functioning of the pancreas or malabsorption issues. Much in the news these days is the widespread increase in diabetes. However, the exocrine function of the pancreas is rarely mentioned, but just as important for survival. This exocrine area and the impact on nutrient deficiencies and metabolism is the book's major focus.

This book can provide you with:

- Practical steps to help heal your body.

- Crucial medical tests to consider for earlier pancreas damage diagnosis, particularly for exocrine pancreatic insufficiency.

- Important health and preventative maintenance medical tests to consider, some of which are not widely known.

- Hundreds of downstream pancreas damage symptoms, some perhaps unexpected, grouped into logical categories.

- Food, water, supplements and medicine to consider for healing.

- Information and actions to help lower bodily insults, inflammation and oxidative stress.

- Information on potential root causes of pancreas damage, vicious cycles and snowball health impacts.

- An example of what happens to the body when metabolism breaks down due to nutrient deficiencies, causing many common modern ailments, and possible actions to take to help restore balance.

Purpose of the Book

Pancreas damage, especially exocrine related, can easily be misdiagnosed or not caught early enough. There is very little useful, practical information for a sufferer with pancreas damage, such as exocrine pancreatic insufficiency (EPI) and the hundreds of consequential symptoms. Please use this book as another data input on your quest to feel better, as it may contain elements of explanation, and potential tests and treatment avenues to consider with your doctor.

It can be helpful to anyone with chronic ailments, fatigue, pain, malaise, low energy, or inflammation. There is a wealth of information here for those suffering from intestinal issues like microbiome dysbiosis, bacterial or yeast overgrowth, irritable bowel, food sensitivities, reflux, malabsorption or nutrient deficiencies. It can be especially useful to anyone with undiagnosed, suspected or even confirmed pancreas damage such as atrophy, diabetes, or exocrine pancreatic insufficiency. EPI can also be linked to other ailments such as hormone imbalances, low testosterone, depression, anxiety, ME/CFS, heart rhythm and breathing issues, and even paresthesia or bone density issues.

Many doctors have not had the experience, and are often too specialized to recognize the problem because of the wide variety of symptoms. Most do not have the necessary time to delve into root cause analysis. They might even be somewhat restricted in providing potentially useful advice, as it might not be approved by their medical board or affiliations. I believe that there are many people who go through years of misery and some even an early grave, either by their body giving out or suicide, without ever getting their exocrine pancreas function diagnosed as a possible culprit of a huge list of subsequent health issues.

Therefore, this book is also meant for doctors with patients who are tough to diagnose with many seemingly unrelated symptoms. Family practice, functional, holistic or integrative medicine doctors, as well as those focusing on life-extension, chronic pain and fatigue, can hopefully use the book as a reference. It is also meant for doctors with patients who have any type of pancreatic damage, such as the gastroenterologists and endocrinologists of the world. Pancreas damage is just one possible illness avenue to check with your patient, as it might be able to help shed some light on an area that is not easily tested for, nor widely recognized. My hope is that you can utilize this book in your practice to spot pancreatic damage earlier and to help those patients with actions to try.

The reason I wrote this book was because I wish there had been something like it available when my health started to decline, without a clear explanation. Especially when I had finally decided to go to a doctor, and another, and another, and twenty more with no results and a rapidly declining situation, the information I am sharing here could have saved much pain and suffering. My single goal in the last six years was to get my life back, and go from being bedridden with no hope of a future, to a functional human being again. I want to share my hard-earned knowledge and the practical steps I took in the hope that it can help people who are dealing with similar quality of life destroying issues. To provide a little helping hand for those struggling to find answers.

But before I delve into my story, let me provide a little background information on a few key concepts like EPI, pre-EPI, CFS, and the crucial organ which started this whole journey in the first place; the pancreas.

The Pancreas

The pancreas is a roughly fifteen centimeter (~six inches) little j-shaped organ that lies sandwiched behind the stomach and the top level of the lumbar spine. There are two major areas that this little sensitive organ, that I did not even know existed before all this, is crucial for.

Endocrine: The function of the pancreas which handles the balancing of blood sugar levels in the body through the production of insulin and glucagon. It also produces hormones such as somatostatin and pancreatic polypeptide. The islets of

Langerhans are clusters of various endocrine cells which produce these hormones in the pancreas.

Exocrine: The rarely mentioned, but just as important, area of the pancreas. The exocrine acinar cells secrete pancreatic juice into the duodenum via the pancreatic duct. Pancreatic juice contains bicarbonate, produced by the duct cells, to neutralize the acidic and partially digested food coming from the stomach. It also contains digestive enzymes, produced by the acinar cells, in order to break down fats, proteins, and carbohydrates into usable nutrients. Without these we would, like I was, slowly starve to death.

What is EPI?

Exocrine pancreatic insufficiency (EPI) is a condition which occurs when the acinar cells in the pancreas are damaged or the organ is unable to deliver pancreatic juice in sufficient quantities, and at the right time, into the small intestine. The main enzymes the pancreas produces are grouped as follows:

- **Lipase:** enzymes that break down fats, such as pancreatic lipase, cholesterol esterase, and phospholipase.

- **Protease:** enzymes that break down proteins such as elastase, carboxypeptidase, trypsinogen and chymotrypsin.

- **Amylase:** enzymes that break down carbohydrates.

EPI causes maldigestion and malabsorption of food. This causes malnutrition and nutrient deficiencies, which in turn impacts the metabolism and metabolic pathways in the body, and subsequently can cause hundreds of downstream health effects. Some known causes of EPI are pancreatitis, infections, cancer, cystic fibrosis, duct obstructions, surgery, or atrophy.

People suffering from EPI are the perfect example of biochemistry in practice and how our metabolic pathways stop functioning properly without optimal nutrient levels. Usually it is not diagnosed as EPI until there is a considerable, roughly 90% reduced, enzyme production and distribution issue.

What is Pre-EPI?

Pre-exocrine pancreatic insufficiency ("pre-EPI") is not an official diagnosis, but a term that I propose to call partial exocrine damage. Just like pre-diabetes for the endocrine side, pre-EPI is where the exocrine side of the pancreas is partially damaged and not functioning optimally. This could be anything from 1-90% less production and distribution of enzymes than is normal and healthy. So, even though a situation might not get an official EPI diagnosis, this still impacts the body's nutrient absorption and metabolism. It can subsequently cause many health issues, albeit slower to result in symptoms or outright breakdowns. The threshold of insufficiency which would actually impact someone's health will of course be different per person.

Pre-EPI is something that is flying under the radar of current medical practice, from diagnosis, knowledge and understanding, to resolution. It is likely a bigger cause of underlying chronic ailments these days than it is given credit for. The lack of sensitive enough and affordable testing tools makes this tough to measure. There is no simple and cheap test available yet, unlike pre-diabetes for which there are a few simple tests to perform.

My suspicion is that malabsorption and pre-EPI are also some of the causes of many classic and premature aging symptoms. If fewer pancreatic enzymes are produced or are available to break down food, it slowly causes nutrient deficiencies with subsequent aging effects. Those interested in life-extension or anti-aging processes should also take a close look at the effect of pre-EPI on aging, and perhaps even consider supplementing with pancreatic enzymes. Many symptoms described later are a good example of how I was aging rapidly and prematurely, including lower bone density, mitochondrial dysfunction, hormones, nitric oxide and testosterone production issues, joint pains, inflammation, difficulty healing, and oxidative stress.

Even food sensitivities and allergies, inflammation and chronic pain can be attributed to improper digestion of food particles, for example, by causing autoimmune reactions or excess toxic byproducts from bacteria and yeast dysbiosis.

What is ME/CFS?

It is chronic, has a wide range of symptoms, and is very difficult to diagnose and treat. ME/CFS is short for myalgic encephalomyelitis (ME) and Chronic Fatigue Syndrome (CFS). Other names used include chronic fatigue and immunity deficiency syndrome (CFIDS), systemic exertion intolerance disorder (SEID), myalgic encephalopathy, or post viral fatigue syndrome (PVFS). It is often misunderstood, as the 'chronic fatigue' label almost sounds benign, or a mental state, and does not do justice to all the symptoms people are suffering from. In the book 'CFS' or 'ME/CFS' are used interchangeably.

Exocrine pancreatic insufficiency (EPI) is another possible underlying cause of ME/CFS with a big overlap in symptoms. Symptoms can include chronic fatigue, weakness, pain, post-exertional malaise (PEM), neurological issues, cardiovascular, issues, motor impairments, immune symptoms, gastrointestinal problems, and mitochondrial dysfunction, to name a few.

It is sometimes a category you end up in when doctors cannot specifically explain the reason for your symptoms. The potential causes for ME/CFS are large and varied, from viruses, bacteria, fungus, chronic stress, chronic toxic exposures, autoimmune, microbiome imbalance, metabolic issues, mitochondrial dysfunction, and unknown causes. Exocrine pancreatic damage, with either pre- or full-blown EPI, is in my opinion an underreported but common cause of ME/CFS these days. The long lasting impact of EPI on metabolism and mitochondrial functioning from nutrient deficiencies is often overlooked, and root causes and bodily insults that cause oxidative stress, mitochondrial dysfunction and microbiome imbalances are frequently not addressed, to the detriment of the sufferer.

Pancreas, the Canary in the Food Supply

The pancreas is the proverbial canary in the coal mine of today's modern food supply and eating habits. It sometimes takes decades before the damage starts to really show, as it is often a slow and stealthy decline. More than a third of the population in the United States has pre-diabetes or diabetes now. It is the same essential organ, so if damage has occurred on the endocrine side there is a good chance there is damage on the exocrine side as well. I read reports that mention between twenty-five and fifty percent of those with diabetes also suffer from exocrine pancreatic damage. This could potentially mean millions of, mostly undiagnosed, people slowly damaging their health and suffering without knowing the underlying cause.

How many news articles and studies mention the various increasing deficiencies of key vitamins and minerals in people these days? How many more cases of diagnosed pancreas inflammation, both chronic and acute, are there these days? Even pancreatic cancer has seen steep inclines. The few times you hear about famous people dying of it is just the tip of the iceberg, and most are often diagnosed much too late. Just look at the massive increase in sales volume of the various brands of pancreatic enzymes over the last decade, and you can get an idea of the steep inclines in pancreatic damage. And those are only the ones that have actually been diagnosed.

The way in which two completely separate medical specialties have split the responsibilities of the same organ is also causing many diagnoses to be missed. The endocrinologist who is specialized in the hormone side of the pancreas does not even think about the exocrine side. The gastroenterologist who specializes in the digestive side of the pancreas does not focus on the endocrine side. And yet the chance of overlapping issues due to similar root causes of this one important organ is sadly overlooked due to this medical specialty split.

The pancreas is a very sensitive organ, and one for which a transplant is an extremely difficult journey. According to my doctors, there is little chance of the acinar cells of the exocrine side of the pancreas to regenerate when extensively damaged or atrophied. Of course the degree of damage per person varies due to the obvious reasons of genetics, epigenetics, differing exposure to environmental stresses, geography, and most importantly, differing eating habits and length of dietary abuses.

Exocrine pancreatic damage is very difficult to diagnose in differing stages of damage through a simple medical screening process. Even when the damage is extreme, as it was in my case, it still took several years to diagnose. Others might still produce much more pancreatic enzymes, but not at a completely healthy level and thus are not digesting their food adequately. Perhaps there is an issue with just one specific enzyme since there are quite a few that the pancreas produces. It is at this time difficult to determine accurately.

The body tries hard to compensate, and it can take a long time to get to a diseased state. Slow deteriorations and initially unnoticed nutritional deficiencies follow. Over time, with continued hits to the organ, this damage spiral can increase, and with it further nutritional deficiencies, microbiome imbalances, oxidative stress, and a subsequent myriad of health symptoms. Some of the damage is initially masked through the intake of multi-vitamins and other supplements, fortification of foods, and even eating larger and more frequent quantities of food. This certainly helped hide my primary health issue for a while.

In hindsight, with the information I had to learn the hard way and am sharing here, it was obvious what was happening to my body. The body is an amazing mechanism that tries very hard to keep everything in balance (homeostasis) despite the bombardment it receives daily through polluted air, toxins in the water and environment, chemicals exposure, unhealthy food and drinks, etc. My body was providing hints many years prior to the complete breakdown, but I just did not know how to read them. Neither do most doctors, who are not focused on preventative maintenance, are trained to attack symptoms in their silo of expertise, and understandably do not have time to delve into root cause analysis.

Supplements and discussions about inputs and outputs of the body are rarely on their radar until it is far too late.

I hope that the next few chapters will help provide you with some practical information from someone who has gone through exocrine pancreatic insufficiency to the point of starvation, breakdown of the body to ME/CFS, and near death. When it was finally diagnosed there was just a sliver left of the organ, barely visible on the scan, and I had less than 10% pancreas function left. In the next few chapters I will share with you what symptoms to look for, what diagnostic tests to ask for, what food and supplements to consider, and what steps to take to reduce the harm to the pancreas in order to start the healing process and hopefully turn your life back around.

The book is split into a few sections, so you can just jump to those which might be of interest for your situation. When you have so little energy it can be tough to even read a paragraph, I know. If you just want to hit the main action items to try to improve your situation, please jump straight to the last chapter.

The usual disclaimer:

Let's be clear, I am not a doctor and nothing in this book should be considered as medical advice. Instead, as my MD brother called it, I am an "experience specialist".

I do not have any affiliation with, nor do I receive any incentives or monetary benefit from any of the information I have written about in the book, including any of the mentioned books, articles, supplements, doctors, medicines, laboratories, companies, etc.

This is my personal experience, which is just an n=1 situation. It is in no way some double-blind tested, scientific review. However, if I can help point just one other sufferer or doctor in the right direction by sharing my anecdotal but hard-earned experiences, as well as the results of my own successful trials and errors, this book was worth writing.

In a nutshell, these are the chapters' goals:

Chapter 1: My Story

How I ended up here and unwillingly, but in order to survive, became a pancreas damage "experience specialist". My "been-there-done-that" story. Perhaps some experiences seem familiar, but have not been considered to be related to pancreas damage. Some actions I took might not have been considered by you or your doctor at this time.

Chapter 2: Symptoms

A reference chapter describing the hundreds of ensuing symptoms I encountered due to pancreas damage, split into logical groupings. You might recognize some you or your patient are suffering from and did not think of them as even being pancreas damage related. It contains large data tables.

Chapter 3: Root Cause Hypothesis

Thoughts on the root cause of my pancreas atrophy and exocrine pancreatic insufficiency. It is a critical look on modern food, water quality and bodily insults causing chronic health damage.

Chapter 4: Tests and Diagnosis

A practical list of tests to ask your doctor about, which can provide information on pancreas damage, related symptoms, nutritional deficiencies, CFS, SIBO, Candida, toxins and preventative maintenance

Chapter 5: Supplements

Supplements to consider by area of concern. It is based on my trial and error experience and collected over the years from many different sources, doctors, research studies, etc.

Chapter 6: Food and Water

Actions to improve food and water quality intake to help your body heal, as well as stem some of the insults that might have caused pancreas damage in the first place.

Chapter 7: SIBO, Candida, and Reflux

Actions to discuss with your doctor for diagnosis and treatment of areas that are linked in their causes, overlapping symptoms, and their resolution steps. Those with pancreas damage can suffer from one or all of these.

Chapter 8: Road to Recovery Actions

A list of action steps to consider, which took me from death's door to a functioning human being again. Included are the major areas to focus on. It contains practical and hopefully helpful information for anyone trying to support the body in its healing, no matter what stage of pancreatic damage or (pre-) EPI.

Appendix: References

A list of additional sources of information. I cannot thank enough the many authors and sharers of info that is easily accessible through the wonder that is "Dr. Google". Without access to this information I would not be alive today.

CHAPTER ONE

My Story

A loosely chronological story of my experience, from deterioration to death's door with no hope, to diagnosis. It shows improvement milestones, the path of learning to uncover the cause, healing steps, and how to become a functioning human being again.

Perhaps some experiences seem familiar to you and were never thought of as related to pancreas damage. Perhaps some of the actions taken have not been considered at this time by you and your doctor.

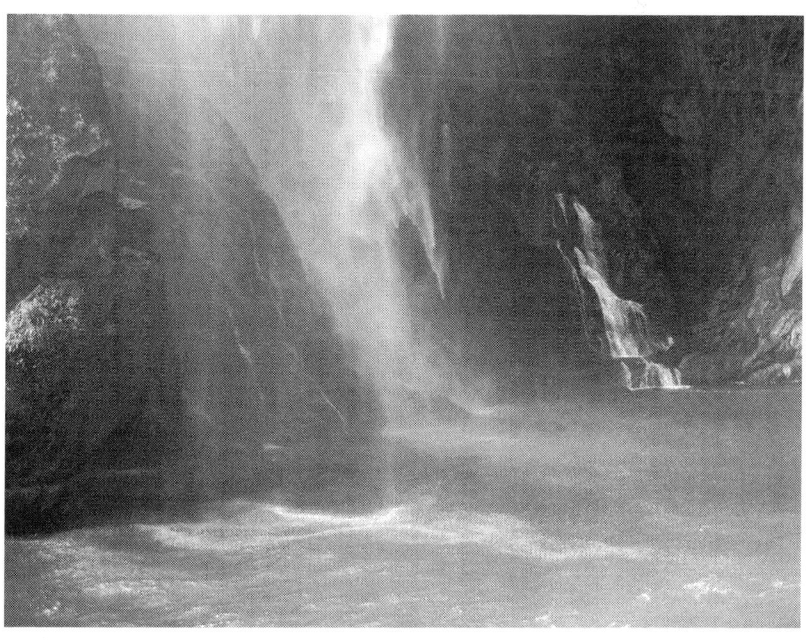

There are so many stories these days of people suffering from chronic modern ailments that are hard to pinpoint and do not get the root cause analysis that they deserve. The age in which previously uncommon or old-age related conditions like exocrine pancreatic insufficiency, diabetes, arthritis, low hormones, autoimmune, etc. are hitting people is getting younger. Combine that with the decreasingly short available time you have with a highly specialized doctor who hardly gets any training on nutrition, supplements and preventative care, along with the massive influence of big business interests, and you have a recipe for disaster.

If you are reading this you are likely living through a similar story, or should I say nightmare, and have been to many doctors without improving your quality of life. You are perhaps still unclear as to the cause of your issues and what to do to get your life back. With what I know now, all of my health issues were in some way related to damage to the pancreas! Key to remember is that there is light at the end of the tunnel, hence me being able to share with you the steps I took to turn my health around.

I have kept the chapter somewhat chronological so you can see the progression of health deterioration over time, with the hints my body was sending me, my experiences with the symptoms, doctors, tests, and improvement steps.

Mine is another story of at first a slow, almost indiscernible declining health, followed by sporadic unexplained health issues, which towards the end rapidly accelerated into eventually my body breaking down. I finally ended up in the emergency room of the hospital one night with numbness (paresthesia) in limbs, unexplained weight loss, weakness, heart and breathing issues. After an active, athletic, healthy, non-alcoholic, non-smoking, non-drugs lifestyle, ending up with not being able to function as a human being was a shock. I was no longer able to work, and had many of the classic CFS symptoms, constant debilitating fatigue, malaise and pain. I ended up homebound for several years and bedridden for many months. In the three years *after* the emergency room low point, the best part of my day was being unconscious. And even that often was not an escape, as sleep would be violently interrupted by panic attacks, breathing and hormone problems, reflux and pain. Every morning I would wake up with the hope of any glimmer of improvement, only to be constantly disappointed. On many days death would have actually been a relief. But, let me start at the beginning.

The Good Times

I was born in Holland to parents who were very aware of the impact of healthy food and the dangers of sugar. From a young age I was always very active and played a variety of sports from soccer and martial arts, to windsurfing. In my early twenties I completed an internship with a management consulting company in the United States and fell in love with a Californian beauty. I was hired full time after graduating and moved to Los Angeles for a travel-intensive career. This meant living in hotels and for many years eating all my meals in restaurants and office cafeterias. No matter where I was, an hour of sporty activity per day and usually ordering the "healthy" alternatives on the food menu was standard. Weekends were filled with social activities and many hours of sports.

First Warning Signs

During all these years I always thought I was living a healthy lifestyle and was thoroughly enjoying it. However, as I now realize, I was terribly unaware of the dangers of the standard modern Western food and water supply, with its excessive sugar, GMO, herbicides, chemicals, industrial oils, and highly processed content. I was slowly but surely chipping away at my health.

The very first hint was how everything tasted super sweet to me in the United States. Everything from milk, bread, cereal, sauces, soups, salad dressings to restaurant meals and even sodas seemed far sweeter than what I was used to. Over time my taste buds desensitized to it somewhat, but in hindsight that was a clear warning sign.

After having lived in the United States for a little over a year, and as much as I hated going to a doctor, I actually saw a gastroenterologist. My stomach felt irritated and the tops of my fingers, near the nail's matrix, were a bit swollen and red. Signs of moderate subacute chronic inflammation in the small intestine and chronic active gastritis due to helicobacter pylori in the stomach were found. The usual antacid and antibiotics were provided, which helped the symptoms, and I continued with my life. Some of the blood tests showed high triglycerides (170 mg/dL) and low HDL (31 mg/dL) cholesterol. My triglycerides-to-HDL ratio was 5.5, when a healthy ratio is less than 2! Root cause analyses of gastric inflammation, food quality intake, stool outputs or important blood test signals were not covered, nor did I have any understanding of what those tests meant at the time.

When I traveled back to Holland, friends and family noticed that I had gained a little weight and my face had filled in more. But, since I had always been quite skinny, this was seen as a positive thing. I just chalked it up to getting older, not a side effect of inflammation. This was also around the time that I would get intermittent annoying mid-back pains and sometimes stitch like pains in the left upper quadrant of my abdomen. Injuries from kickboxing or soccer happened easier and took longer to heal.

During most of my twenties I felt invincible. Work hard during the week, party on the weekend, with sports usually every day and extra on the weekend. I could eat or drink anything without any visible or perceived impact, or sensitivities. But, at some point my energy level started to stutter. I would get tired more easily and did not have as much cardio during soccer or beach volleyball games. Alcohol, which had only always been a weekend evening social thing, was no longer tolerated as well. I thought the main cause was the standard sixty to eighty hour work weeks and constant plane travel that was the main cause of my energy dipping. But, it was such a gradual thing over time that I did not really pay too close attention.

Coasting Along

In my thirties another hint from my body that something was not quite right was my stool. Now, this is a less salient topic so if you just had breakfast, perhaps come back to it later. But it is very important, and something doctors, especially primary care or gastroenterologists should pay more attention to. I had to go more often per day, it became softer over the years, and it turned more yellow brown than the normal deep brown. The smell intensified and at some point I would have to take my shirt off to go, otherwise the smell would stick to the shirt. It would also stick to the bowl more, so that the toilet brush had to eventually be used every time I went. I know now that if you have to wipe too much, something is not right. It means that there is either something wrong with the food intake or your digestion system, and you are not digesting fat and thus not absorbing food properly. Look, if it happens occasionally or if you have traveled and need to get accustomed to different food that is normal. If you ate too large a quantity, or too rich a meal, and were not able to produce enough enzymes to break down the fat that time, this happens. It becomes a concern when it is more than a one-off. With me this was also a slow progression that went in spurts, because the atrophy of my pancreas slowly became worse over time. In hindsight, logically there was a correlation between the amount of energy I had and the quality of my stool, as I was not getting all the nutrients from my food.

In addition, almost every cholesterol test that was done over the years in my thirties showed low HDL, increasing LDL, high triglycerides-to-HDL ratio, and slowly increasing fasting glucose levels. Never was I a big drinker, only on weekends with friends, but I became more and more intolerant of alcohol, and eventually I completed stopped. I also became lactose intolerant, where a single coffee creamer or M&M would set my stomach off very noisily.

The Wheels Start Coming Off

When I turned forty the wheels started wobbling much more, even though I had drastically changed my work life balance to no longer have to travel much, nor live in hotels during the week. Although I was married to an angel of a wife, lived in a cozy apartment with our furry son, had no immediate financial worries and had no obvious reasons for it, I was becoming depressed and apathetic. I had less and less energy and desire for talking or meeting up with friends and family. My wife and I used to travel for vacations regularly, but that petered out completely. I thought that perhaps I was just getting older and not exercising enough, but I could no longer muster the energy to work out as much either.

I decided to see an endocrinologist due to the low energy, low libido, mood swings, irritability, memory issues, mind fog, slow healing joint injuries, and a troubling twelve pounds muscle weight loss in two months. Blood tests confirmed a vitamin D insufficiency (25.7 ng/mL), low HDL (41 mg/dL) and elevated LDL (139 mg/dL) cholesterol levels, low-normal testosterone (Total 513 and free 8.4 ng/dL), on the high side of normal estradiol for a male (38.2 pg/mL), slightly elevated hemoglobin A1c (HbA1c 5.4%), and low aspartate aminotransferase AST (13 IU/L).

The recommendation was to take vitamin D supplements and that was it. There was no discussion as to why my testosterone was lower, nor any mention of its link to vitamin D. There was no looking into why my vitamin D was so low, and even by the wide standard endocrine ranges it was low. Low AST levels were ignored even though I now know that it can be tied to a vitamin B6 deficiency. There was no talk about food, or any additional nutrition related measurements, even though in hindsight those numbers were a clear warning. I was unknowingly continuing to do damage to my body throughout this time.

This was around the time I had to stop with Thai boxing due to injuries not healing. A simple pull-up exercise gave me golfer's elbow that no amount of physiotherapy would heal. Jogging would hurt my knee and hip. Windsurfing had become impossible on most days and even a tiny cut on my fingers would give me a staph infection that my immune system could not handle. This happened frequently and required antibiotics multiple times.

My back would give out intermittently from a simple movement, not even when weight was involved, and I would find myself on the ground having to wait for the spasm to subside. If I sneezed I had to be careful not to throw my back out, and getting in and out of bed required a very specific set of movements. No matter how hard I tried, I could not gain muscle back, and felt like I was getting softer and fatter. Now keep in mind that I was still skinny, or should I say "skinny-fat", which is likely another reason why no alarm bells were going off with any doctor. Outwardly I may have looked trim and healthy, but my fat was the worst kind; visceral. And, skinny does not necessarily mean healthy!

One Year into Deterioration

The vitamin D supplementation helped quite a bit. In addition, I was taking a strong multi-supplement, containing minerals, vitamins, and phytonutrients every day, which helped delay the inevitable. However, things were still not getting back to where I was hoping to be. I would get unexplained infections of the prostate and urinary tract, with blood in my urine, again requiring antibiotics. My mid-back issues became more frequent and I went to see a sports medicine chiropractor who helped me walk out a few times when I came crawling in. Even the sports massage therapist noted that the muscle tightness and cramping in that mid-back area was not normal, and pointed to a few vertebrae that started sticking out more in that same area. Interestingly all the back problems were around the same physical level of the body where the pancreas is located. Perhaps another hint from my body? I often read about people having a nagging lower back pain that is hard to determine the root cause of, and often thought to be mechanical. Few have likely thought about pancreas damage or nutritional deficiencies as a possible cause.

Two Years into Deterioration

To still get a little workout I would use an elliptical machine or stationary bike, and simple exercises like push-ups and sit-ups. However, I now started to get chest pains, but not the classic post-exercise muscle ache. Also, I started getting a deep and constant rib pain which would wrap around to my left shoulder blade. Exercise would exacerbate it. It never completely went away and would fluctuate in intensity. I felt out of breath much quicker and had far less energy than normal for sports or fun. Foot cramps, which can indicate mineral deficiencies, were frequent, and I would sporadically get swollen lymph nodes in my armpits. Since it worried me a bit I went to see an internist, who had a chest X-ray and ultrasound done. But, the results did not provide any answers. In hindsight this was related to nutritional deficiencies such as CoQ10, magnesium, vitamins B2 and B6.

Low Testosterone

Low testosterone is something you are bombarded with through commercials these days, as it is common place now and at a lower age as well. My testosterone had dropped further (Total 357 and free 6.9 ng/dL), which is close to deficient even by the standard range, and certainly unhealthy for my age. What is not often discussed is that it can be just another symptom of too much sugar, nutritional deficiencies, pre-diabetes, diabetes, or exocrine pancreatic insufficiency. Zinc, B and D vitamins, and omega-3 fatty acids are all required by the body to produce testosterone. So, if you are deficient in any of those, they will get used in higher priority areas of the body. The body is smart enough to determine that procreation is less important than, for example, keeping the heart ticking or the brain functioning.

For a few months I tried testosterone replacement gel, which did raise my testosterone temporarily to the mid-to-high 500s (ng/dL), but it also raised my estradiol to 87.5 (pg/mL) at one point. A healthy ratio of total testosterone to estradiol (T/E) in males my age is between 30 and 40, yet mine was around 7.

Generally I did not feel much better, and would get occasional dizzy spells and bouts of vertigo when lying down. So, after a couple of false starts with compounding pharmacy versions as well as a patented one, I stopped all together with experimenting with hormone replacement therapy (HRT). It made me feel worse.

This is one of those frustrating and sad areas where you see a myriad of big budget advertisements and high dollar testosterone replacement therapies to attack a symptom. People are not looking at an important root cause of low testosterone, namely nutritional deficiencies and diet. But, you cannot patent nutrition and diet! I can trace the decline to a low of 349 (ng/dL) total testosterone and <6 (ng/dL) free, until my EPI was diagnosed. The improvement started when my nutritional deficiencies turned around along with diet, supplements and pancreatic enzyme replacement therapy. Without testosterone replacement and without much exercise I increased my testosterone by 80%, to a perfectly normal level! Even though this topic is a bit male centric due to my personal experience, I would expect a similar nutritional impact with female hormones and testosterone levels in females.

But, I am getting ahead of the story timeline.

Silent Reflux

This was also around the time when acid and silent reflux symptoms like post-nasal drip, morning hoarseness, a lump in the throat feeling, tender esophagus even during breathing, constant throat clearing especially after eating or drinking, dry coughing, and some stabbing pain around the heart area started to become really noticeable. I started watching my intake of tomato sauce, coffee, spicy food, chocolate and mint, but this did not really help much. Starting in my thirties, I rarely drank alcohol and was never a smoker. The rare soda would really flare up throat and chest irritations. A couple of times I had woken up in a panic as it felt as if I could not breathe, which subsided when sitting up. In hindsight this was stomach acid making its way up. Another strange symptom was that if I turned my head with food or drink in my mouth, it would go down the wrong hole. This started to happen much more frequently.

Finally, I decided to see another doctor, a gastroenterologist, as there was just a gut feeling that there was an issue with my stomach, intestines and digestion. I had also noticed intermittent blood in the stool and a higher frequency per day that I needed to discuss with him. He performed a sigmoidoscopy, where a portion of your colon is checked with a camera. He also completed an endoscopy with biopsies to look at the esophagus, stomach and part of the duodenum. No issues were found. I was told to use an acid blocker (Prilosec) for two weeks and put, of all things, more fiber in my diet. All the other symptoms, including the big weight loss, stool issues, hormone and nutrient imbalances were ignored.

When I look at a couple of the pictures from the procedures in the report now with my untrained eye, I notice what looks like red, irritated tissue and some very unhealthy looking yellow stool. But what did I know? This was still the time when I completely and blindly trusted and believed everything a doctor would tell me, without questioning it or performing my own research.

One of my doctors went much further, and tested for food allergies, checked the functioning of my thyroid the proper way (Including T4, free T4, T3, free T3, reverse T3, TPO and TG antibodies), checked for celiac disease and did a Lyme disease panel. No issues were reported. Lipids were also tested again, and although slightly better than before, were still showing unhealthy ratios of triglycerides-to-HDL and higher LDL levels. One other anomaly that was ignored at the time, as it is mostly only looked at if too high, was a low alkaline phosphatase ALP. Now I know that it can be a sign of malnutrition, pointing to possible deficiencies in vitamins B and C, zinc and phosphorous. Low ALP can be linked with fatigue, shortness of breath, temperature sensitivity and weight loss, all of which I had.

Commencing Breakdown

Three years into the deterioration, and at this point I was still in denial that things were falling apart. I thought of all the various symptoms as standalone items instead of part of a complete picture. The first half of the year I still forced myself to continue with work as usual, do as much exercise (really very little) as I could muster, and started planning a trip to Hawaii. Perhaps it really was all just in my head.

My back went out badly again and I nearly piled down a staircase, and had trouble standing and walking because of it. I decided to see a spine specialist who had really helped out my wife in the past. This was also the time when I started getting paresthesia of the hands, fingertips, feet and left knee. Most of the paresthesia was a numbness feeling, as if those areas had gone to sleep. Sometimes it was a feeling of ants crawling, or strange electrical zaps and burning sensations. My joints started crackling and aching quite a bit, and I had more frequent neck pains and headaches. After MRIs and X-rays were done of both the lumbar and cervical spine, the results showed some degenerative damage, but nothing out of the ordinary for someone my age. There was no visible impact on the nerves.

At this time panic was starting to set in because I was feeling so unhealthy. It felt like I was wasting away without any explanation. I could barely drive myself to the doctor and felt unsafe doing so. The spine doctor was very patient, supportive and referred me to an internist and neurologist, as none of my nerve symptoms were spine related. He also asked me whether there was something else going on, hinting at drug or alcohol abuse and psychotherapy. A fair question, although this one stung since I had always led such a clean lifestyle, drugs-free, smoke-free, and with some social alcohol in my twenties and early thirties. He set me up with physiotherapy to strengthen the muscles that had atrophied, which was one of the reasons my back kept seizing up.

In addition, I felt a lot of bloating, distended belly and intestinal pressure that felt like it was pushing into my lungs. My stool, which at the time I still did not recognize as being an issue, had become even more yellow, bulky, smelly, floaty and sticky. Going to the bathroom ten times a day and never really feeling relieved was normal for me now, and I had to plan around knowing where bathrooms were. Now I know it was due to malabsorption, too quick an intestinal motility and steatorrhea symptoms tied to exocrine pancreatic insufficiency. I could no longer break down fat properly. Sometimes I would see undigested bits of food, other times it would explode to powder when flushing, and infrequently it was diarrhea looking stool. If you have any nutritional deficiencies or stool disorders (anything that is not a smooth chocolate brown sausage that does not leave a mark, like shown in the Bristol Stool Chart) it could mean that you are not breaking down food properly in your stomach and intestines. You do not have to have a pool of fat floating on the surface of the toilet water in order to think of pancreatic insufficiency, as I never had that. If you are going five to ten times per day this is not normal.

Complete Breakdown

Halfway through the year is when everything came to a complete and rapid breakdown, when I could no longer function nor push myself through the symptoms with pure will. My energy level had still been declining, I had lost another ten pounds of muscle, I was nauseous most days, started getting panicky feelings for no reason, had trouble sleeping, had hypoglycemic bouts, would get micro-dizziness where the room would spin briefly, became quite sensitive to heat and cold, had strange itchiness spells, even worse mind fog, terribly blurred vision, etc. I developed more and more sensitivities to food which I had never had before, for example, tomatoes, coffee, tea, tomato sauce, cucumber, chamomile, apple, fish oil, krill oil, yoghurt, peppers, black pepper, paprika, flaxseed, casein, Brussels sprouts, cabbage, gluten, and turnip. Vitamin C and magnesium pills would cause stomach and intestinal issues.

One morning, silly me, I thought I could swim in the cold water in the bay to feel better, and nearly drowned after less than ten minutes. I had trouble breathing, was close to fainting and barely made it to shore, even though it was only thigh-high water. In tears, and I am not an emotional person by any means, I stumbled home with the realization that things really were not okay and I could no longer pretend. That evening the weakness and numbness in my hand prevented me from even holding a fork in my left hand without it falling to the floor. Simple coordination issues and clumsiness became a daily thing, something I had never had before.

The paresthesia became much worse and it now included my lips, back of the head, both hands, a few fingers, left arm, left knee, ankle, elbows, both feet and some toes. Sometimes the numbness would wake me up from sleep, when the whole side where I was sleeping on would have no feeling for a while. I would get weird sunburn sensations on various parts of my body, including my eyelids, even though I had not been in the sun. Sometimes my hands would feel as if dunked in snow for minutes, and start tingling. The fingertips of my thumb, index and middle finger and the outer edge of my hand were numb on most days. Strange shooting pains in feet, limbs and head, and involuntary twitching of muscles and neck spasms would happen randomly.

There were months when it felt like I could not get enough oxygen, even though I was breathing normally and did not have a respiratory infection. It would even wake me up from a deep sleep sometimes. I would have to lie down with my head out on the balcony, gasping for air like a fish out of water. It was quite scary when I could not absorb enough oxygen. This feeling should not be confused with a panic attack or hyperventilation, which is quite different. It is more like trying to breathe through a thick, heavy blanket and I felt oxygen starved. In hindsight, this was likely an important signal of secondary mitochondrial dysfunction. For a few months prior to the EPI diagnosis, I used an asthma inhaler that provided temporary breathing relief.

My physiotherapist stopped the treatment for my back as she felt it was too dangerous. All of my life my blood pressure was healthily low, but now it would swing wildly. My heart would skip beats, I would get dizzy, get instant headaches, and be out of breath from the simplest of physical therapy exercises. Even the numbness in my limbs would increase sharply during the therapy sessions. In addition, I had made no progress in months from these sessions, and was moving like a ninety-year old man.

It finally hit me that things really were not okay and I had to cancel all my current and future work projects. This was tough to do since I was self-employed, with no other means of income and no safety net. Luckily, I had saved up enough to be able to pay the growing and very high medical bills. Any planned trips were cancelled and I became homebound.

One evening in June I finally had my wife take me to the emergency room, as I had never felt this bad in my life. For my weakness, shortness of breath, paresthesia, heart palpitations, chest pains and tightness, a CT scan of the chest with dye was made. It all ended up with no clear diagnosis and was told to see a pulmonologist for my lungs and a cardiologist for my heart. Interestingly, almost two years later, another gastroenterologist noted that there was barely any pancreas left to see on the emergency room CT scan. But, it is difficult to find a doctor that would immediately link my symptoms to the pancreas, so it was not even on the radar at the hospital. I did not even know what a pancreas was, where it was located, or what it did at this time.

The Wheels Are Off

In the next few months I continued getting weaker, lost more weight, was nauseous every day, had more frequent dizzy spells, panic attacks from sleep, night sweats, pain breathing, and shortness of breath. I felt like a zombie with no energy. Everything felt surreal and I suffered from constant fatigue, brain fog, blurry eyesight, night blindness, lack of concentration, confusion, memory issues, constant anxiety, jittery-yet-so-tired feeling, emotional lability, irritability, and many layers of pain as well as a debilitating malaise. My mind would start playing tricks on me, and I would randomly smell odors like smoke that were not there.

There were moments where my mind fog was so thick I could not understand sentences spoken by my wife or on television. I could not digest the information quickly enough and would get confused. I would even catch myself stuttering and have dyslexia when trying to speak or type an email, something I had never had in my life.

The hormonal imbalance was such that I could not watch most television programs as I would get a panic attack from certain sounds or events on a show. I was in constant fight or flight mode, and had that stomach churning nervous feeling all the time. Constantly being in fight or flight mode is fatiguing and wears down the adrenal glands, especially when you are low on nutrients.

For quite a few months even sleep would not provide me with relief anymore, as I would wake up more often in a sweaty panic with numb limbs, or with a lack of oxygen feeling. There were many nights where every hour or so this would happen. In hindsight, this was due to hypoglycemia. My blood sugar level would get too low and cause an adrenaline dump to wake me up. Other times this was due to sleep apnea, where I would stop breathing until I was startled awake in panic as I was getting low on oxygen. It is amazing what the body subconsciously does to stay alive, with all its various continuous monitoring and rebalancing mechanisms that we are normally not even aware of, until things start breaking down.

I found that lying on my left side would make it harder to breathe and would kick in heart palpitations. Standing up was easier to breath, but for many months I just did not have the strength to stand. Even sitting up at some point was tough. On and off I would get bouts that sometimes lasted a few minutes, sometimes months, where my heart would skip every third or fourth beat and felt like it was flip-flopping in my chest. My heart rate would at times dip into the low twenties beats-per-minute. Sometimes it would stop for what seemed like five to ten seconds at a time with subsequent dizziness and confusion. One vivid moment was when my heart had not kicked back in for what seemed about ten seconds, and everything suddenly felt super quiet, eerily so. After I slid off the couch and banged quite hard into the table, a jolt of adrenaline kick-started my heart to race for a while, before going back to its "normal" premature ventricular contractions (PVC).

I did not have the energy to speak or interact with people. No longer did I have the strength to do regular life activities. Eating was torture, sleep was broken, walking up the stairs felt like climbing a mountain, and taking a shower was tough. On top of that, the relentless layers of pain, malaise and fatigue were soul-sucking and I was holding on by a thread. I would get massive long-lasting bruises from the simplest bumps, or just even lightly rubbing my nose, or a blood draw. The things you normally take for granted were gone, such as being able to understand a conversation, say a few words, pick up a utensil to eat, not be nauseous during eating, being able to walk instead of shuffle like a ninety-year old, ride a bike, drive a car, being able to watch television or enjoy music, easily remembering the names of your friends and family members, a day without pain, enjoyment in anything, etc. You get the idea; my body was breaking down.

It is sadly just one of those things that people around you, including doctors, friends and even family members will not comprehend unless they have gone through something similar themselves. You are just one of many for the doctor, who logically needs to take an emotional distance, and due to the system of "sickcare" has very little time for you. Colleagues, friends and family members have their own lives and struggles to attend to. You will find out who your true friends are but you will have no energy for them, nor will they be able to provide day-to-day support. This is not anyone's fault. It is just the reality of being chronically ill, and it is lonely. Before the diagnosis my wife even became fed up with my unexplained lack of energy, the mood swings, the depression and apathy. I broke down in front of her not knowing how to communicate how ill I felt. But she is a ride or die kind of girl. If not for my amazing wife taking care of me during these years with mental, emotional and physical support, driving me to doctors, grocery shopping, cooking, getting medicine, loving embraces, all the standard life things you take for granted, and just being there for me, I would not be alive today.

Trying to Understand

This was the start of the roller coaster ride of seeing doctor after doctor, performing test after medical test, all the while getting worse and not getting any answers. Some quotes from doctors that I wrote down along the journey:

"Your pancreas is fine"

"It is not an endocrine issue"

"I do not think it is something pathological"

"What would you like me to do?"

"Perhaps you need to consider a psychiatrist"

"There is nothing you can do to reduce the inflammation. I can prescribe you painkillers, but you will just become addicted and end up killing yourself."

"Why do you want to do an MRI of the abdomen?"

The information in the next few chapters would have been particularly helpful after the twentieth specialist still had no diagnosis, forget about even a glimmer of a root cause or potential solution, and I felt like I was close to death.

Dr. Google became my friend, and I spent all my waking and somewhat alert hours and energy on reading and researching. Anything I could come across in various languages, no matter how technical of a paper, or fluffy of a product-selling website. If any of my symptoms were mentioned, I would try reading it and take notes on what tests I wanted to have done. Some illnesses I wanted to cross off were really far-fetched, but many symptoms were so common. Since I would forget otherwise, I would prepare a list of discussion points, symptoms, tests to do and diseases to cover, and take this with me to every doctor's visit. These notes also helped me to be able to write this book years later. I had kept track of how I felt most days, what I tried in terms of food and supplementation, as well as interesting bits of information I gathered during my reading.

Like many of you reading this, my situation had stumped a few dozen doctors with varying specialties, after countless ECGs, Ultrasounds, X-rays, MRIs, CT scans, blood, urine and stool tests.

We looked for rare genetic diseases, autoimmune diseases, cancers, tumors, sexually transmitted diseases, many common bacteria and viruses, many Lyme disease co-infections, allergies, parasites, heavy metals, chemical or mold exposures, genetic markers, most of the CFS related diseases, and neurological disorders. Nothing came out that would explain my situation.

Our apartment was tested for mold, moisture, indoor air quality, chemicals and even electromagnetic fields (EMF), all with good results.

Some of the medical doctors and alternative therapists I saw included:

- Pulmonologist
- Cardiologist
- Lyme disease specialist
- Thyroid specialist
- Immunologist
- Rheumatologist
- Gastroenterologists (multiple)
- Pancreas gastrointestinal surgeon
- Functional or integrative medicine specialists
- Orthopedic surgeon and spine specialist
- Internal medicine specialist
- Endocrinologist
- Neurologist

- Vascular specialist
- Primary care or family practice physicians
- Physiotherapist (Physical therapist)
- Psychiatrist
- Amino acid specialist
- Acupuncturist
- Energy kinesiologist
- Sports medicine chiropractor
- Allergist

Four doctors mentioned specifically that my pancreas was absolutely fine. One stated that my issues were not pathological, and two others even suggested looking into Prozac and a psychiatrist! I am censoring my true reaction here, but "yes doctor, I am depressed because I feel like I am dying and no one is able to help me". To be fair, they all wanted to help but lacked the experience and skillset in diagnosing and treating exocrine pancreatic insufficiency. It just illustrates how difficult pancreas damage is to recognize and diagnose.

Glimmer of an Explanation

One evening my wife suggested taking a magnesium supplement, and I very quickly felt a positive impact. That night I had not slept better in many months. This strengthened my suspicion that many of my symptoms pointed towards malnutrition and malabsorption.

There is a test by SpectraCell which checks for nutrient levels within white blood cells that caught my attention during one of my internet searches around malnutrition. Luckily, I found a local doctor who does that test at his office. With the help of this functional medicine doctor, additional blood, stool and urine tests, including detailed nutritional and organic acid ones from specialized labs like Genova Diagnostics, Doctor's Data and Great Plains Laboratories were ordered. These tests pointed in the direction of nutrient deficiencies, mitochondrial dysfunction, neurotransmitter imbalance, pancreatic enzyme deficiencies, malabsorption, small intestinal bacterial overgrowth (SIBO),

Candida yeast overgrowth, and intestinal microbiome dysbiosis. Sadly, these tests are not common practice and most insurance companies do not cover them. More on these key tests in a later chapter, but why would this happen when I thought I ate a healthy and balanced diet without many vices at all?

Finally, after I was quite adamant on wanting this test done, an MRI of the abdomen uncovered the underlying cause of my hundreds of symptoms and side effects. Over 90% of my pancreas was gone through advanced fatty atrophy ("spectacularly atrophied" according to a surgeon) with subsequent exocrine pancreatic insufficiency (EPI) causing malabsorption, malnutrition, nutrient deficiencies, breakdown of body and organ functions, secondary mitochondrial dysfunction and eventually Chronic Fatigue Syndrome.

Now, you could have differing levels of damage, atrophy or malfunction of the pancreas, whereby you are just not producing the necessary amounts of pancreatic enzymes for a healthy life. The effects could be very subtle with slight nutritional deficiencies and take a very long time to notice. Or it could be a more extreme case like mine, which clearly showed up on the MRI.

One of the tests done later was the stool elastase test. It can help determine whether you have EPI, but often after the fact, and I am not convinced it is all that accurate. Elastase is an enzyme produced only by the human pancreas and is not influenced by taking pancreatic enzymes. During my worst months my elastase showed only a slight insufficiency (194 µg/mL versus >200 being normal). It was not until a year after my diagnosis, when I was on pancreatic enzyme replacement therapy (PERT), that the elastase level really dropped into the 30s (µg/mL). Since then it has been fluctuating wildly. More recent tests, years after the diagnosis, showed increases by more than 100 (µg/mL).

Another common test that was done is the 24-72 hour stool fat test (Fecal lipids), which checks to see how much undigested fat is still in your stool. Anything over seven grams for a twenty-four hour period is considered an indicator for EPI. However, you are expected to eat one hundred grams of fat per day during the test, which is a tough one when you feel so ill. My results were just below seven grams per twenty-four hours, but I barely ate fifty grams of fat during the day as I was so nauseous at the time. It clearly showed I was not digesting fat properly, but it provides no information on the other enzymes that the pancreas secretes.

Here is the danger. Most people will likely not have their pancreas show up as atrophied as mine on an MRI, if they can even persuade their doctor to order one. In addition, the absolutely amazing nutrition and urine organic acid tests are not on most doctors' radar. Therefore it is very difficult to determine whether you have pre-EPI or full-blown EPI until it is much too late. There is no easy blood test available, and there is no easy way to see whether your pancreas is secreting enough of any specific enzyme. Is it fat, carbohydrates or proteins which are not properly digested, and at what levels are enzymes missing? This is currently not possible to do as one standard test, which is a clear gap in current medicine. For the endocrine side of the pancreas it is super easy to determine whether you have insulin issues. The HbA1c, glucose and insulin tests can tell you whether you are pre-diabetic or full-blown diabetic.

It would not surprise me at all if there are way too many people who suffer and die painfully without the exocrine damage of the pancreas ever being discovered as the root cause of their myriad of health issues. I very nearly gave up myself in order to escape the downward malaise and pain spiral.

Chronic Pain

One element of feeling debilitated is a chronic level of pain and malaise. For me there were layers and layers of pain, and it was not until one pain was resolved that suddenly another pain would now came to the forefront. Pain would range from random sharp stabbing, tearing, pressure, the doubling over seizing type, to dull or irritating. It would vary in various areas of the body from deep between the ribs, lower- and mid-back, behind the shoulder blade, head, neck, muscle, leg bones, foot, front and back area around the pancreas, stomach, small and large intestines, colon, plexus, flank, chest, toothache, etc. Skin pain would be frequent to the point where a usually very pleasant, slightly warm, ocean breeze would hurt. During the recovery period it was like peeling an onion. For instance, the pancreas area pain would lower, only to have an intestinal or bone pain now become more noticeable from the white noise of constant pain.

I refused to go down the road of painkillers and its subsequent side effects and addiction, even though I did receive some from the doctors. Pain is a signal from the body that something is wrong and requires healing. Painkillers do not resolve the root cause but mask this signal. High dosage Ibuprofen I tried for two weeks, which not only did not help with the pain, but it exacerbated things. Grin and bear, with sleep, Epsom magnesium baths and meditation, as well as the occasional aspirin or acetaminophen was about as far as I was willing to go. Of course, everyone's pain level and how you experience it is going to be very different, just be aware of the pitfalls.

One of the debilitating elements was the constant complete body ache and malaise that usually you only get when you have the flu with high fever. It seemed to me that my body was signaling that something was wrong and I needed rest and repair. As you might know, it is not a bacteria or virus that causes pain. But, it is your own body's response via, for example, the release of cytokines which forces you to curl up in a corner so that it can try to heal whatever damage is going on.

You might recognize some of the differing pains and not have realized it was a subsequent effect from pancreatic damage. There is a summarized list in the symptoms chapter. But, there was not a single day in the last four years without pain, and it would not surprise me if many of you out there have suffered far longer.

I watched the documentary film about Tim Bergling, better known as Avicii, the late great Swedish EDM DJ. It captures him suffering through pancreas damage, pain and malaise. Sadly, I recognize that stooped-over-in-pain, gaunt look of his. Likely, his pancreas damage was recognized much too late, and he did not have the necessary integrative, holistic guidance from the very start of his health troubles. He passed away much too young!

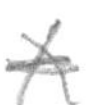

Low Point and Suicidal Thoughts

When there is no light at the end of the tunnel. When your day consists of nothing but weakness, pain and misery, your thoughts go from hopelessness and despair, to thinking about suicide, and then to actually planning it. I started to think of ways to get final relief with the least impact on loved ones and innocent bystanders. One very bad day was actually when my wife had driven me to a pancreatic specialty hospital in Los Angeles, and we were staying on the sixteenth floor of a hotel nearby. This was years into a still declining health, after having seen many doctors and specialists, and with no end in sight. The pain levels were so high I was doubled over. I had been nauseous for about six months and could barely tolerate any type of food. The surgeon at the hospital had no idea about the cause, impact or solution of exocrine pancreatic insufficiency. He said he could write a prescription for the pain, but I would become addicted, and that there was nothing that could be done to lower inflammation. Since in my mind this was the last resort doctor's visit, it was disappointing. Now, I do not blame the surgeon since his training likely did not cover it, but I had expected more from an institute specialized in pancreatic diseases.

Whilst my wife was at work after the visit and I was back at the hotel, I spent a good thirty minutes contemplating launching myself off the balcony. You know that toe-curling feeling when you are standing at the edge? However, even though I was really looking forward to the relief, all I could think of was the impact on my wife of having to identify the remains, as well as the people that might witness the aftermath.

But, the reason for me sharing this unpleasantness is that I am still here, and I was able to turn my health and life around. I very nearly gave up in order to escape the pain and malaise. But, no matter how low you get, please at least try the things I am sharing in this book. The good news is that there is light at the end of the tunnel even though most days you will not feel that there is a way out. You can slowly get more minutes of relief, followed by hours, followed by days. You will have dips here and there, so there will always be that lingering doubt of when you will get smacked down again. Know that the road to recovery takes time and requires patience and dedication, but take comfort in any of the tiny positive increments. Continue reading the other chapters to find out about medical tests to help determine possible causes, and steps you can to take to help get back on the road of healing.

Do not lose hope!

Off the Ledge

After the abdomen MRI results came back, the functional medicine doctor referred me to a gastroenterologist who finally diagnosed the exocrine pancreatic insufficiency (EPI) due to advanced fatty atrophy of the pancreas. You can also see it sometimes referred to as non-alcoholic fatty pancreas, since such damage is more often seen with alcoholics. But clearly, significant pancreatic damage can also be caused by the modern Western diet impact, with subsequent long term high triglycerides and oxidative stress.

The functional medicine doctor and gastroenterologist split the duties respectively along the lines of supplementation and pancreatic enzyme replacement treatments, in the hope of improving my situation.

Nutrient Supplementation

Without supplements, EPI is not something you can function with. They are absolutely required to recover from the various deficiencies and subsequent cascading health effects. I would not be sitting here writing this without the support of supplements. Luckily, we live in a time when every conceivable supplement is available at a touch of a button, to be delivered to your doorstep. The functional medicine doctor provided me with many insights into reputable supplement companies and types of supplements to try, from oral or injectable, to slow intravenous drips.

To give a few examples, using magnesium and B-vitamins resulted in immediate improvements of some symptoms by easing those deficiencies. Some of the massive and relatively quick improvements were around my paresthesia and asthma-like symptoms, which disappeared within a couple of months. All the feeling came back to my limbs and digits, and I no longer needed the asthma inhaler to catch a breath! I felt the oxygen being used properly again when breathing in. Vitamin K was now clearly being replenished, as I no longer would get the massive bruising after a simple blood draw. Hypoglycemia and related nightly panic attacks improved drastically. Blood pressure spikes and the inability to sleep well were resolved with magnesium. The complete lack of coordination and things like the inability to hold a fork were resolved. The brief, but very scary, heart stoppage episodes were resolved. Vitamin D levels improved slowly, and the immediate effect of supplementing it was an improvement in my mood. Other areas saw a much slower improvement, especially around energy levels, intestinal issues, neurotransmitters, malaise and pain, but they required additional steps as you can read further down.

Another significant boost came from feedback from a friend of the immunologist I had seen, who specializes in mitochondrial dysfunctions. It is what two doctors now suspected as being an issue. He recommended a mitochondria supplement cocktail of CoQ10, vitamin B1, creatine, and L-carnitine. Within five days my heart palpitations, which had been ongoing non-stop for over four months, were gone completely!

This led me to find another very helpful book with great explanations linking mitochondria dysfunction to Chronic Fatigue Syndrome. Based on the book I added D-ribose and nicotinamide riboside, and had a few vitamin B complex injections. My functional doctor also had a few mitochondria support supplements to try such as MitoThera, CorvalenM and ATP Fuel. All these supplements brought about a big jump in improvement. In hindsight, malnutrition and the nutritional deficiencies caused a secondary mitochondrial dysfunction. If you look at the Krebs (a.k.a. citric acid) cycle, which shows the body's main energy production metabolic pathway, there are some crucial nutrients needed to keep it, and the mitochondria, functioning properly. This includes magnesium, iron, manganese, zinc, copper, CoQ10, vitamins B1, B2, B3, B5, and C, lipoic acid, D-ribose and amino acids such as arginine, and L-carnitine. If L-carnitine is lacking, fatty acids cannot get into the mitochondria and metabolize. Obviously, fatty acids supply will also be a problem if the pancreas is not providing the enzymes to break down food in the first place. L-carnitine can also help lower LDL cholesterol. The important take away is that just one specific nutrient deficiency can escalate into one or more of the various cogs in the machine becoming dysfunctional.

CoQ10 deserves a special mention. Much later I experimented with it some more and confirmed that it was the absolute key in resolving all my heart issues. I must have become so deficient in my tissues and organs that it had impacted the functioning of my heart, and been a big factor in the secondary mitochondrial dysfunction. It was confirmed when I read in another great book by a cardiologist, the importance of CoQ10 along with magnesium, L-carnitine and D-ribose on the functioning of the heart. This was something the cardiologist I had seen a few times for all my heart issues was utterly clueless about, as his talking points were pacemaker, cardiac ablation and statins. As a side note, it also helps me with pancreas area pain, which I take as a signal I need to supplement CoQ10 a bit more.

Keep in mind that just adding supplements to the mix is only part of the solution. An even more important step is to immediately start with pancreatic enzyme replacement therapy (PERT).

Pancreatic Enzymes

Maldigestion is an impaired breakdown of nutrients through either lack of digestive enzymes and/or gastric acid production issues. This in turn causes malabsorption, as nutrients are not broken down into useful absorbable components, which then causes malnutrition. With EPI, you are slowly and painfully starving to death, first nutritionally and eventually completely. Your muscle tissue and bones are used up internally as nutrient fuel. This is when pancreatic enzymes come into the picture.

Pancreatic enzymes are absolutely crucial for survival when you have EPI, and can also help those that have "pre-EPI". I was prescribed pancrelipase called Creon, which is one of a few prescription brands of pancreatic enzyme replacement pills. They are essentially pancreatic enzymes such as lipase, amylase and protease from a pig's pancreas in tightly controlled quantities.

There are also many over the counter digestive and vegetarian type of enzyme supplements containing, e.g., bromelain and papain. But, this is not something I would use regularly because of how crucial it is to get very specific and controlled amounts of enzymes for each meal. It might be helpful in addition to the real deal, but not instead of. This is not something you want to gamble with!

Initially I took a low dosage of 24,000 units as if it was a vitamin pill, not understanding how it worked. This was also the time where my stomach was so irritated with gastritis, likely because of imbalances in the mucosa layer, SIBO and Candida overgrowth. My intestines were completely inflamed and I was nauseous all the time. In the hope of lowering the stomach burning and pain I stupidly lowered it to 12,000 per meal, but at least now I understood it needed to be taken with the meal in order for me to be able to digest the food.

Overall things were not that much better, even though some big symptoms had been resolved. Instead I felt in some ways like I was still getting worse. This is where proper guidance from a doctor who truly understands EPI and all the additional interrelated health effects would really have helped. It is one of the reasons for me writing this book, in order to help patients, and doctors with helping any future patients.

Simply prescribing some pancreatic enzymes, although absolutely vital, is just not enough!

The amount of enzymes taken is crucial and it takes some trial and error to get right. Even how you spread the pills during the meal makes a difference, all of which I had to learn the hard way.

After five months of this, on top of which I was now taking nausea medication in order to force down food, I decided as a last resort to travel to a pancreatic specialty institute in a world renowned hospital. One of the gastroenterologists had recommended I triple my enzyme intake, spread the pills during the meal, and that I should not restrict my diet in any way. At this point I was clutching at straws, so anything that could possibly help I grasped on to as a mental life line. Increasing the amount of enzymes was a life saver though, and I would suggest erring on the side of too much as opposed to too little in the beginning. You might have to adjust the levels over time and I have since increased the amount further to between 72,000-108,000 units per meal. Please keep in mind that this amount varies per person, and the quantity and type of food consumed.

Gluten, SIBO, Candida Yeast, Silent Reflux

Three months later I had stumbled across a great book on the negative health impacts of wheat and gluten. I started with a gluten-free diet even though I did not have celiac disease. Since most wheat products strip out the healthy wheat germ for increased shelf-life, you are left with mostly starch, which is sugar or glucose to the body. This helped especially with hypoglycemia, inflammation, stomach bloating and intestinal pains. Throughout this time I tried many different supplements, acupuncture treatments, vitamin injections and vitamin drips, and continued with a variety of tests. I was also doing things like meditation, yoga breathing, magnesium salt (Epsom) baths, and infra-red sauna sessions to help with handling the pain.

Yet another three months later and I read about all the potential negative impacts of Candida yeast overgrowth and small intestine bacterial overgrowth (SIBO) on health, including such symptoms as malabsorption, gastritis and nausea. This was likely also the cause of my silent reflux this whole time. In hindsight, it is logical that excess sugar and carbs in the diet, in addition to EPI and an already imbalanced microbiome, allowed an excess of creatures in areas where they normally should not flourish. The esophagus, stomach and duodenum should be quite clean, without much yeast or bacteria. Ever seen what yeast does when you add sugar to it? Just imagine that reaction happening in your stomach, with stomach acid bubbling up into your esophagus. So, at this time I asked my functional medicine doctor to help me address Candida overgrowth. I started with Nystatin antifungal for at least a month, in conjunction with natural antimicrobial drops and supplements which attack the biofilm. Now I was starting to see some improvements.

To also tackle the silent acid reflux, I inclined my bed a good ten inches at the head to avoid acid flow up during sleep, and tried a low acid diet for a month so that my esophagus could calm down. A digestive enzyme called pepsin comes up into your esophagus during reflux and it thrives and reactivates on anything acidic. It is supposed to stay in your stomach to help digest your food, not digest your esophagus or throat! I had three weeks of antacids to lower the acid in my stomach temporarily and ease the gastritis, along with some supplements to help soothe the stomach. By lowering the acid from both food and beverage intake, as well as from up-flow from the stomach, it allowed the pepsins to calm down and actual healing to occur in the stomach, throat and esophagus.

Another three months later and I asked my doctor for a SIBO breath test, which confirmed my bacterial methane production in my stomach and small intestines was eight times normal. My hydrogen production levels were normal. It is important to test for both methane and hydrogen as they indicate different types of bacteria. Likely you will be given Rifaximin antibiotics, but this alone is not effective, especially if most of the bacteria are methane producers. I used a combination of Rifaximin and Neomycin for ten days.

Again, another welcome improvement! Especially the nausea, stomach and intestinal pains, burning feeling, bloating, brain fog, concentration, dyslexia, stuttering, memory, confusion, and eyesight blurring issues improved considerably after the SIBO and Candida treatments. I was no longer literally crying in my soup, could once again enjoy and comprehend a bit of television or remember a four-digit pin code for longer than two seconds. I wish I had known all this information many years ago.

Amino Acid Supplementation

To continue with the timeline, it was now more than two years after having taken my first Creon pancreatic enzyme pill and the diagnosis of exocrine pancreatic insufficiency. I was still struggling. Yes, many nasty symptoms had been resolved and blood work was still improving for the most part, but I was still homebound and unable to do more than a bit of part-time work from home, for a very understanding old client of mine. The only time I left the house was to visit doctors and get lab blood draws done. I was still in constant malaise and pain, full body ache and skin pain, something you normally have when suffering from flu with high fever. I still had little energy for anyone or anything, except going for a short walk with the dog and the occasional small bike ride in the neighborhood. I could not gain any muscle weight back. And, I was still apathetic and depressed, and generally did not see much reason to stay alive.

Too stubborn to give up though, I went through another battery of tests and a small car's worth of out-of-pocket expenses to see if there was still something else going on. Every Lyme disease panel and cofactor infection test, any available Chronic Fatigue Syndrome cause test, and any other virus or bacteria test which might have some resemblance in terms of symptoms, were completed. It was interesting to see how many prior virus infections were still detectable, even some from thirty years ago. But, nothing came up to indicate anything current that would explain the symptoms.

My body was essentially telling me that something was still not right and that I needed to rest and heal. Determining what "that" was, was the hard part. I went back to the nutrition organic acid tests. Now that I knew a little bit more, it seemed obvious that I was still not absorbing food properly, especially protein, with subsequent amino acid deficiencies. This seemed to me a logical cause for my pain, malaise, depression and apathy. Without sufficient tyrosine amino acid, your body will not have the building blocks to produce enough dopamine. Without enough phenylalanine amino acid, I could not make enough tyrosine, which in turn would result in the inability to produce enough serotonin. Almost all the amino acids are necessary to produce endorphins, the body's natural painkiller, so if you lack just one you cannot produce endorphins properly. Without enough tetrahydrobiopterin (BH4), a key cofactor in the production of all the neurotransmitters, which in turn requires enough zinc and vitamin B6, I would not be able to synthesize all the necessary elements. So after going down a rabbit's hole with all the bacterial and viral testing, I was back to the pancreatic damage resulting in malabsorption, and just not having enough building blocks for a normal life.

This was when I started experimenting with amino acid supplementation. Going back to a brand my functional doctor had mentioned, but due to all my stomach issues at the time I could not tolerate it then, I started with amino acid multi pills. These contain all the essential and nonessential amino acids. Essential amino acids are those that your body needs every day to function and cannot make by itself, so they have to come from absorbing protein. Nonessential amino acids are those that your body can synthesize, but only when it has enough building blocks and cofactors (vitamins, minerals, metabolites, etc.) to do so.

Wow, all I can tell you is that adding an amino acid supplement to the supplement regiment when you suffer from EPI is an absolute must to consider. It improved my mood, it improved my malaise, it lowered my pain levels and I was daring to hope a little. At this point I found a doctor who specialized in amino acid therapy, to see whether I could learn some more. After a few thousand dollars and a few urine and blood tests more, it just confirmed what I had already found out. The nutrition organic acid test is vital in analyzing any deficiencies, and amino acid supplementation is crucial when suffering with pancreatic damage.

ME/CFS - Chronic Fatigue Syndrome

At some point my body's standard metabolic pathways and enzymes were hindered from functioning properly. Viruses, bacteria, illnesses, nutrient deficiencies, toxic overloads and other insults to my body could have caused blockages and functional hindrances to cause a form of mitochondrial and metabolism dysfunction. Not to mention that my immune system could have been kicked into a constant state of high alert as well. There are many paths to get to Chronic Fatigue Syndrome (ME/CFS), which is why it is such a difficult one to analyze and overcome. I was not born with a mitochondrial dysfunction, so it was a likely result of EPI. As I mentioned earlier, the scariest part was the heart and breathing issues, where it felt as if I was not using oxygen properly to produce sufficient (ATP) energy. Years of weakness, fatigue, pain and malaise can be soul sucking. 'Chronic fatigue', it almost sounds benign, or a lazy or mental state, and not so debilitating. What a misnomer really, as it is so far removed from any of those labels. I would certainly have preferred to have repeatedly broken many bones in my body, and heal from that, than suffer from years of ME/CFS!

Your world can become really small. In my case I went from a happily married world traveler with a successful career, a good social life and a lot of sports activities, to my couch and bed for many months followed by years of homebound suffering. The biggest trips for years were walking around the block with the dog, and that was only after I became strong enough for little walks. Even a little exertion could floor me for days or weeks. With ME/CFS you have no energy for anything or anyone.

This is a tough symptom to describe to those that have not experienced it either firsthand, or as a caretaker. Even close friends and family will not truly understand unless they have gone through something similar, or are taking care of you on a day-to-day basis. There are of course various levels of ME/CFS, from completely debilitated and unable to communicate, clean and feed yourself, to having no energy for life and being in a constant form of pain and malaise, and anything in between. Sometimes you may not even look classically ill, even though you feel horribly ill.

Exocrine pancreatic insufficiency (EPI) or pre-EPI is just one pathway to ME/CFS. After years of nutrient deficiencies and metabolic breakdowns, my body's mitochondria had a tougher time generating energy (ATP), and my metabolic pathways were not functioning as they should, with all the subsequent effects. The weakness, pain and malaise levels fluctuated wildly inter- and intra-day. It is so frustrating, because one minute you can have enough energy to take a shower, and yet an hour later you are unable to have a conversation with your loved ones. I always try to describe the malaise portion as how you would feel with flu and high fever, hungover and with food poisoning all rolled into one, but then imagine that this feeling does not stop for the foreseeable future. You just want to curl up in a ball in a corner and die. I think one of the reasons for the fluctuations in energy is that suddenly mitochondria or some enzymes get enough of a specific nutrient cofactor that it was lacking, and a block is overcome temporarily. As if the engine stutters to life for a bit and then peters out again due to a lack of specific nutrients.

Recovery

It was now three years since my advanced pancreas atrophy and EPI diagnosis, with less than 10% pancreatic function left. After many years, I finally had enough energy to travel to my motherland and start writing this book to share my findings. It had been a journey of six years of unhealth, five years without knowing a pain-free day, four years of non-stop malaise, over three years of being homebound where anything food related, and frankly life itself, was torture. For those of you reading this book and suffering from chronic fatigue, pain or illness, or any pancreatic damage, you have likely suffered far worse.

The pancreas gets into a vicious cycle of damage because of the constant hits through food, drink, excess sugar, chlorinated and fluoridated tap water, plastics, heavy metals, exposure to environmental, herbicide and other toxins, and excess free radicals causing oxidative damage in the body. The lack of nutrients, antioxidants and cofactors hampers the handling of these free radicals and further injures the pancreas. It is also why smoking and alcohol, which produce large amounts of free radicals, are often linked to pancreatic damage.

The pancreas truly is the canary in the coal mine of the modern world, too bad so few are really listening.

Over these years, the notes I kept on how I felt, the doctors' visits, the tests, the research, the trial and error actions and results, I can now summarize here with the hope of helping at least one other person or doctor. All the steps I took which helped me are listed in the next chapters, including elements of food, water, medicine, supplements, reduction of insults, medical tests, lowering of oxidative stress, lowering of inflammation, etc. Hundreds of my symptoms have been resolved by taking these steps, but because I had to uncover and piece together most of the information myself it took a lot longer than it should have.

The good news is that my heart is ticking normally again without any skipped beats, arrhythmia, flip-flopping, or premature ventricular contractions. My breathing has returned to normal and I no longer feel oxygen starved, nor have any asthma-like symptoms. Silent reflux, small intestinal bacterial and Candida yeast overgrowth have been resolved. I sleep normally again without being woken up by hypoglycemia, lack of oxygen, breathing issues, or adrenaline dump panic attacks. No longer am I doubled over in pain for weeks on end. My malaise levels are not even close to what they were before, and many days now I do not even notice. My paresthesia issues, coordination issues, eyesight issues, memory, stuttering and dyslexia issues are all completely gone.

All the layers of constant pain, from nerve, chest, back, bone, skin and intestinal pain have been resolved. My back is much stronger and has not seized up in quite a while. The soft tissue, joint pains and inflammation are gone. Cuts, bruises and sprains heal normally again. No longer am I hunched over and shuffling like a centenarian. Waking up, my muscles no longer ache as if I had run a marathon during my sleep. My testosterone level increased 80% and is normal again. My nutrient deficiencies have been resolved. My microbiome is more balanced and I am able to enjoy food again.

My latest stool test results were good, with normal fat content (on PERT), and even improving pancreatic elastase levels. Elements such as triglycerides, HDL, cholesterol ratios, homocysteine are all normal again. My pre-diabetes has been resolved, and my glucose and HbA1c levels are healthy again, although I do of course have to watch sugar and carb intake closely. No longer am I anxious all the time for no reason. No more panic attacks, and my mood is much more positive. Chronic Fatigue Syndrome symptoms are so much better. No longer does it take days or weeks to recover from a simple exertion. But, I do still have to take a nap and meditate on many days and be careful not to overdo it.

Many of the simple things I took for granted before I became ill I can do again. For example, being able to hold a fork, short term memory, having a conversation, playing with the dog, enjoying a sunset, making my own food, buying my own groceries, chores around the house, enjoying music and television, etc. Most food sensitivities have been resolved and I can eat more normally, although I still have to be very careful of the ingredients, avoid most restaurants, and continue to follow a mostly primal, organic food lifestyle. I am able to do light weights, simple exercises, short bike rides and work part-time again.

The results are night and day and are still improving, having gone from being bedridden with no hope in sight to a functioning human again!

Summary

In hindsight I was suffering from multiple related issues which were hampering my healing. All these key problem areas should have been tested for, addressed and tackled together:

1. Pancreatic enzyme replacement therapy (PERT).

2. Food and water quality.

3. Deficiencies in macro-, micro- and phyto-nutrients.

4. Deficiencies in fatty acids.

5. Deficiencies in amino acids.

6. Small intestinal bacterial overgrowth (SIBO).

7. Candida yeast overgrowth.

8. Microbiome dysbiosis.

9. Silent or acid reflux.

10. Oxidative stress, bodily insults and inflammation.

11. Neurotransmitter balances.

By following the steps I share in this book I was able to resolve almost all of my symptoms, and go back to being functional again.

CHAPTER TWO

Symptoms

This is a reference chapter containing the descriptions of the hundreds of snowball effect symptoms I encountered due to my pancreas damage, split into logical groupings. You might recognize many of them and not realize they were pancreas damage related.

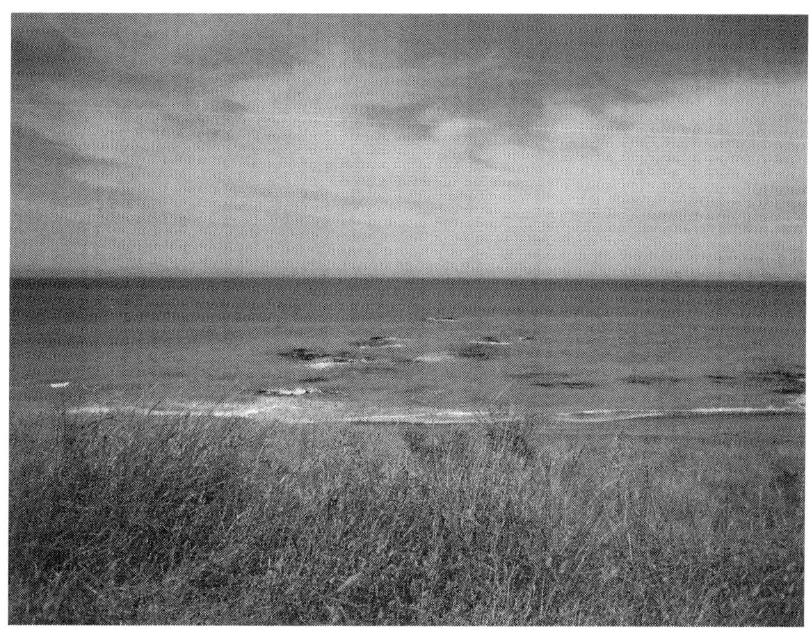

In the prior chapter I covered many of the symptoms in a somewhat chronological fashion, including small sections highlighting symptoms like ME/CFS, acid or silent reflux, low testosterone, SIBO, and Candida. This chapter is more of a reference section. I have loosely grouped the main symptoms I experienced into categories, so that you can check whether there are any familiar ones. In your case, some symptoms may not yet have been suspected to be a subsequent effect of pancreatic damage, microbiome imbalance or nutrient deficiencies, and open up a path of exploration.

In addition, I have listed relevant abnormal urine, stool and blood test results with a few notes, as I consider them possible symptoms as a result of my pancreas damage. Important to note is that my tests are spread over a few years, and results varied over time. Some tests were done at my worst, whilst others were well into the healing phase, showing results of experimentation of food and supplements. Too much fish and olive oil was a good example of one of my experiments showing up on the test data.

Since it is such an important source of information, a separate section shows the nutrition organic acid test results, with explanation notes collected from my Doctor's Data, Genova Diagnostics, and Great Plains Laboratories test results and their guides. Keep in mind that I have only listed those where I had abnormal readings, as there are many more test results provided by those labs.

This chapter is split into the following subsections so you can easily jump to the area which might pertain to your situation or interest.

- **Symptoms by category**
- **Blood tests symptoms**
- **Stool tests symptoms**
- **Urine tests symptoms**
- **Nutrition organic acid tests symptoms**

In hindsight, every symptom eventually could be traced back upstream to nutrient deficiencies caused by pancreas damage, exocrine pancreatic insufficiency (EPI), and microbiome dysbiosis as the overarching medical cause.

Symptoms by Category

The list of my symptoms, imbalanced urine, stool, and blood test results was in the hundreds. Many symptoms can point to a wide range of ailments, which is why pancreatic damage is so difficult to diagnose. Since some symptoms are shared across categories, I loosely grouped them into the following:

Gastrointestinal:
Anything to do with the intestinal tract, from food to stool.

Microbiome Dysbiosis:
Imbalances of the microbiome, including small intestinal bacterial and Candida yeast overgrowth, and too few beneficial intestinal bacteria or too many detrimental ones.

Hormones:
These include energy, testosterone, emotions, sleep, and sensitivity type symptoms.

Neurotransmitters:
Symptoms of various imbalances in neurotransmitters, such as dopamine, serotonin, norepinephrine, etc.

Cardiorespiratory:
Symptoms of the heart, lungs or some combination of both.

Musculoskeletal:
Symptoms of muscles, bones, soft tissues, eyes, and nerves.

Chronic Fatigue Syndrome (ME/CFS):
Mitochondrial dysfunction, Chronic Fatigue Syndrome or myalgic encephalomyelitis type symptoms.

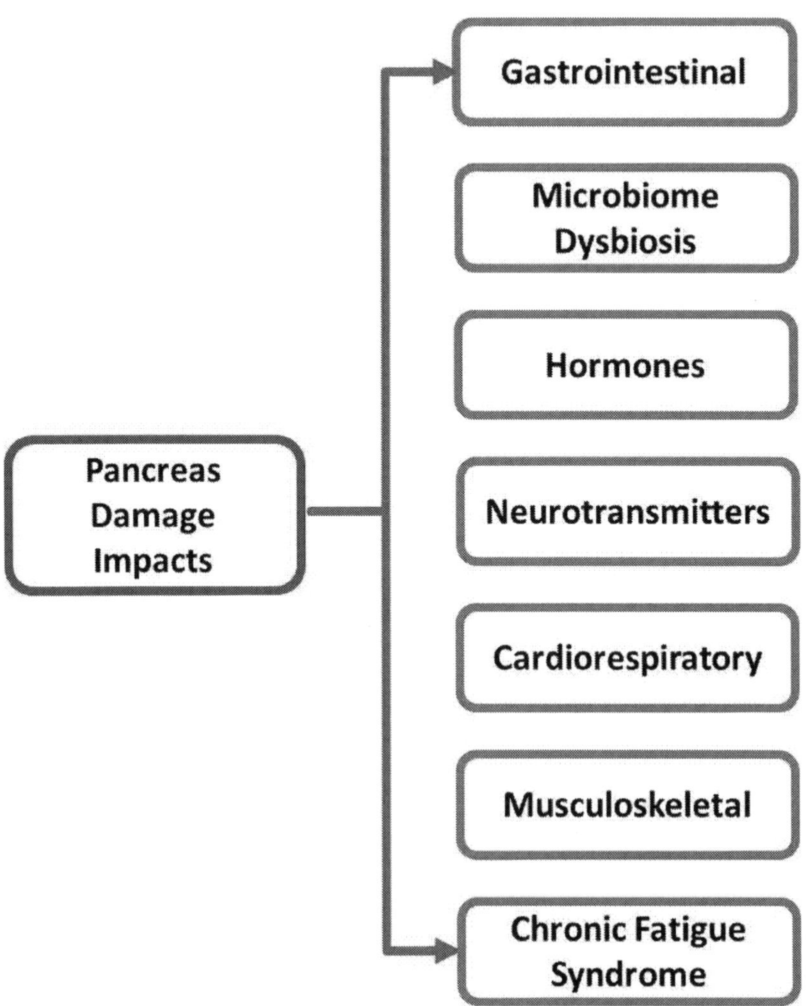
Pancreas
Damage
Impacts
Gastrointestinal
Microbiome
Dysbiosis
Hormones
Neurotransmitters
Cardiorespiratory
Musculoskeletal
Chronic Fatigue
Syndrome

1. Gastrointestinal Symptoms

Blood Sugar Level

- Episodes of hypoglycemia even during sleep
- Wild swings
- Glucose too high
- Insulin too high
- HbA1c too high
- Pre-diabetes

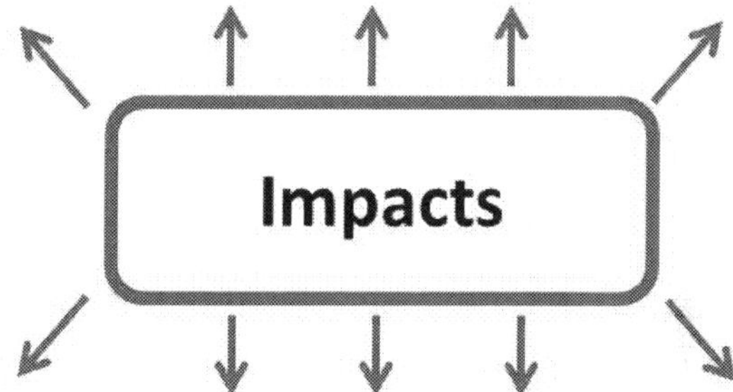

Pain

- Diaphragm
- Plexus
- Flanks
- Stomach
- Intestines
- Pancreas area, deep, front and back
- Stronger after eating
- Gnawing and burning in stomach
- Left side worse

Outputs

- Stool: fatty, yellow, sticky, smelly, explode to powder when flushed, mucus, stringy threads
- Constantly feeling the need to go
- Frequent stool up to 10x per day, 3-5 average
- Blood in stool and urine
- Greenish urine

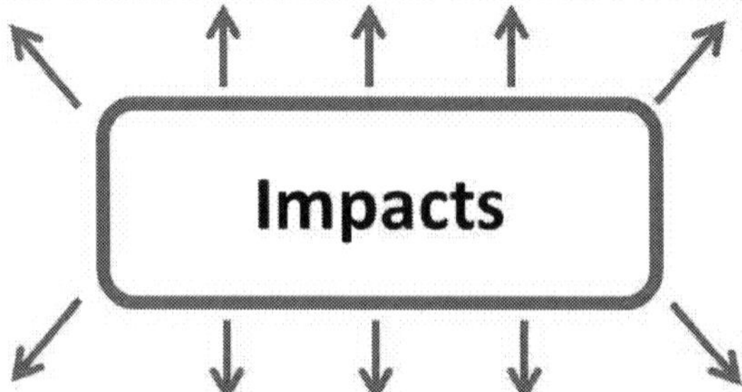

Lipids

- Unabsorbed fatty acids
- Cholesterol LDL too high
- Triglycerides too high
- Cholesterol HDL too low

Imbalances

- Maldigestion
- Malabsorption
- Metabolism
- Secondary mitochondrial dysfunction
- Reduced capacity to metabolize amino acids, carbs, fatty acids
- Microbiome dysbiosis
- No appetite
- Stomach spasms
- Dry mouth, bad breath
- Pancreatic elastase low
- Alanine transaminase (ALT) low
- Alkaline phosphatase (ALP) low
- 1-Methylhistidine high
- Food passage speed too fast
- Oxidative stress and inability to handle excess free radicals

Deficiencies

- Slow starvation
- Micronutrients: vitamins and minerals
- Macronutrients, phytonutrients
- Enzymes
- Amino Acids
- Electrolytes

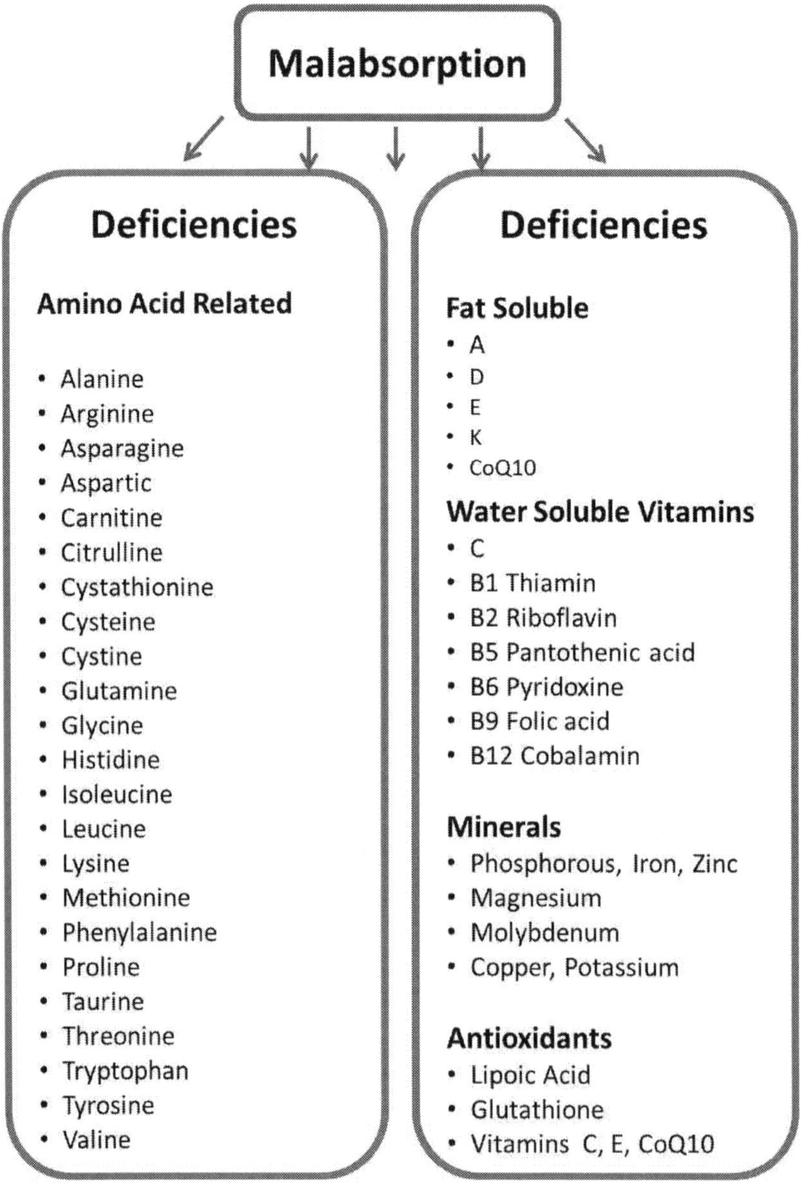

Malabsorption

Deficiencies

Amino Acid Related

- Alanine
- Arginine
- Asparagine
- Aspartic
- Carnitine
- Citrulline
- Cystathionine
- Cysteine
- Cystine
- Glutamine
- Glycine
- Histidine
- Isoleucine
- Leucine
- Lysine
- Methionine
- Phenylalanine
- Proline
- Taurine
- Threonine
- Tryptophan
- Tyrosine
- Valine

Deficiencies

Fat Soluble

- A
- D
- E
- K
- CoQ10

Water Soluble Vitamins

- C
- B1 Thiamin
- B2 Riboflavin
- B5 Pantothenic acid
- B6 Pyridoxine
- B9 Folic acid
- B12 Cobalamin

Minerals

- Phosphorous, Iron, Zinc
- Magnesium
- Molybdenum
- Copper, Potassium

Antioxidants

- Lipoic Acid
- Glutathione
- Vitamins C, E, CoQ10

2. Microbiome Dysbiosis Symptoms

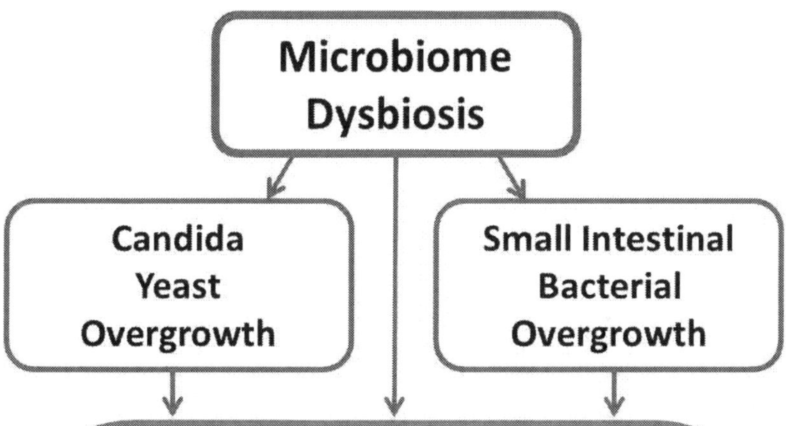

Issues

- Too much pathogenic bacteria and yeast
- Too little beneficial bacteria and yeast
- Intestinal pains, burning in stomach
- Depression, apathy, suicidal thoughts
- Body ache, skin pain, malaise
- Food and smell sensitivities
- Sugar cravings
- Fatigue, mind fog, concentration, eyesight issues
- Irritability, mood swings, anxiety
- Gastritis, nausea
- Diarrhea, irritable bowel and stool issues
- Skin issues: dryness, rash
- Excessive burping after eating
- Bloating, distended belly
- Molybdenum deficiency
- Malabsorption and nutrient deficiencies
- Impaired break down of gluten, lactose, phytates
- Oxidative stress: inability to handle free radicals

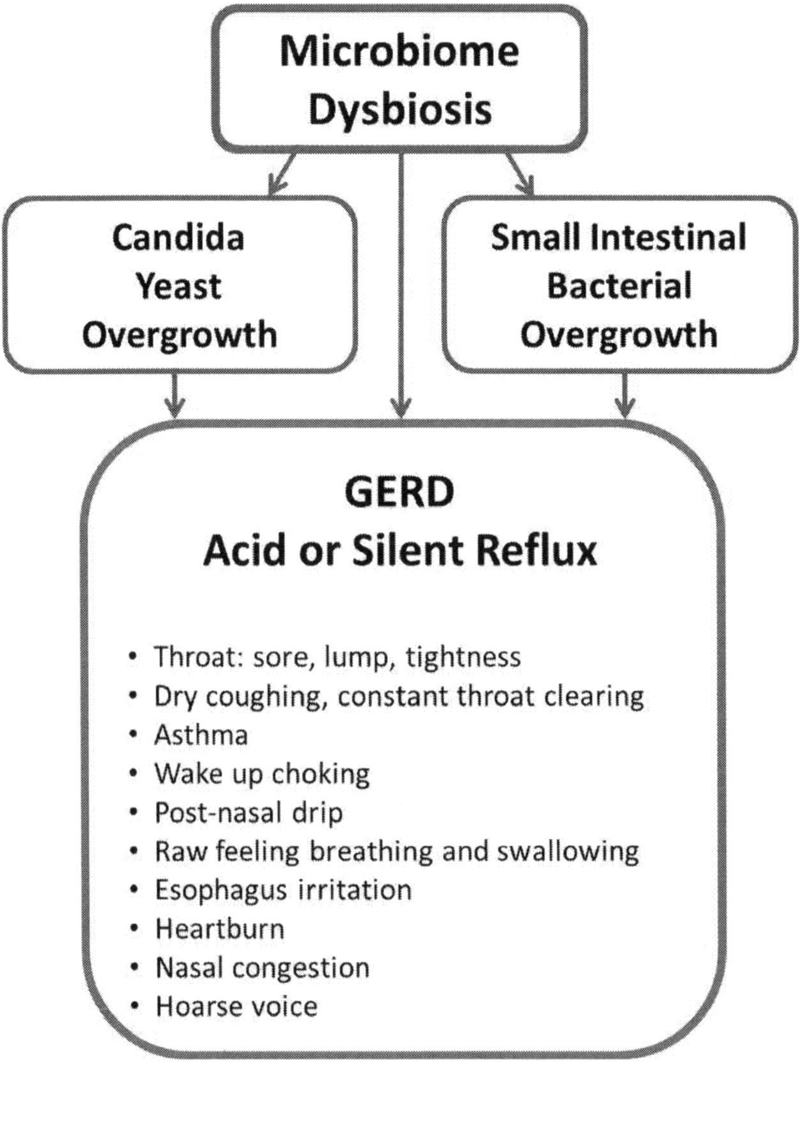

Microbiome Dysbiosis

Candida Yeast Overgrowth

Small Intestinal Bacterial Overgrowth

GERD
Acid or Silent Reflux

- Throat: sore, lump, tightness
- Dry coughing, constant throat clearing
- Asthma
- Wake up choking
- Post-nasal drip
- Raw feeling breathing and swallowing
- Esophagus irritation
- Heartburn
- Nasal congestion
- Hoarse voice

3. Hormones Symptoms

Sleep

- Insomnia
- Not restful
- No longer an escape
- Panic attack wake up from deep sleep
- Excessive night sweats
- Many symptoms are caused by adrenaline and cortisol spikes

Emotions

- Wild mood swings
- Panic attacks
- Anxiety and nervousness
- Constant fight or flight
- Irritability
- Many symptoms are caused by adrenaline and cortisol spikes

Testosterone

- Low testosterone, total and free
- High estradiol
- No libido, no morning glory
- Bone density issues
- Mood swings, fatigue

Energy

- No energy
- Drowsiness
- Malaise
- Flu-like symptoms
- Insulin spikes

Sensitivities

- Sound
- Light
- Cold
- Heat
- Smell
- Food
- Changes in taste sense

4. Neurotransmitters Symptoms

Brain

- Mind fog
- Confusion
- Inability to focus
- Memory issues
- Temporary dyslexia and stuttering
- Smell hallucinations (Phantosmia)
- Issues with absorbing information through sight or hearing

Emotions

- Despair, pessimism and depression (low serotonin)
- Emotional lability
- Suicidal thoughts
- Apathy, exhaustion, inability to get pleasure (low dopamine)

Pain

- Malaise
- Flu-like symptoms
- Skin ache
- Body ache
- Less able to handle pain (low endorphins)

An example of the influences of some of my cofactor deficiencies on neurotransmitters:

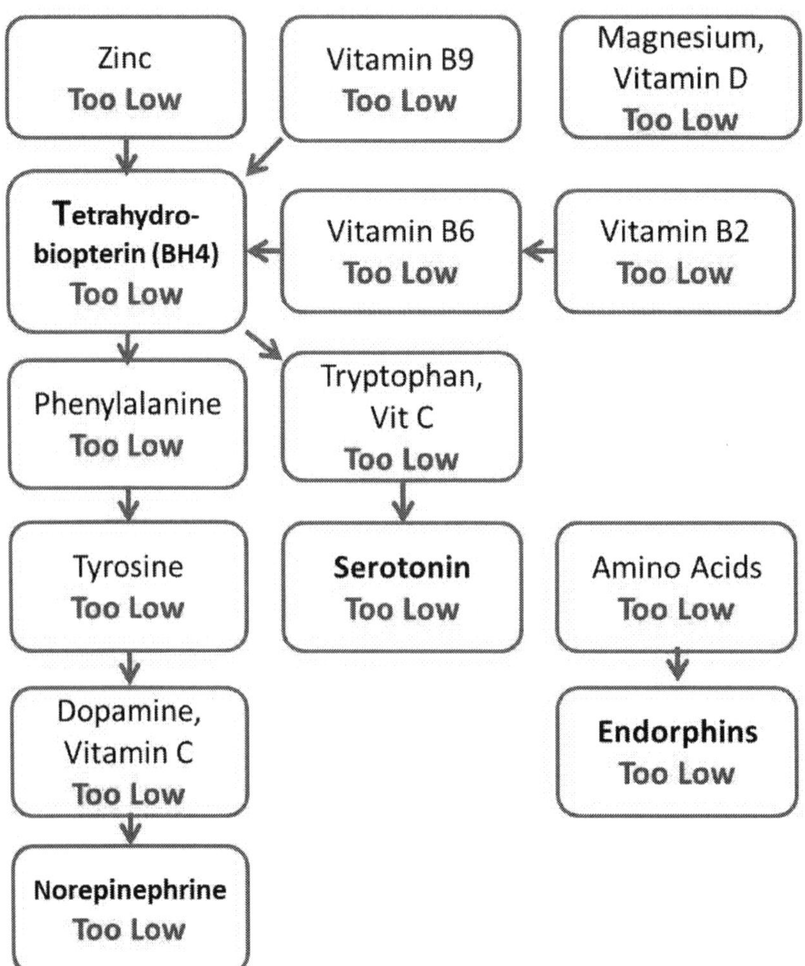

5. Cardiorespiratory Symptoms

Lungs

- Sleep apnea
- Pain breathing
- Asthma-like symptoms
- Air hunger
- Shortness of breath
- Lungs irritated
- Felt like small blockages, pressure, tightness
- Slight wheezing when lying on left side
- Spirometry test abnormally low

Heart

- Palpitations
- Brief and random stoppages
- BPM heart rate of low 20s at times
- Premature ventricular contractions (PVC)
- Blood pressure spikes and drops
- Thumping and flopping
- Racing randomly

Combination

- Vertigo when lying down
- Stabbing pain in chest
- Pressure on chest
- Headaches
- Disorientation
- Dizziness, spinning, near fainting
- Talking is too strenuous
- Standing or sitting is too strenuous
- Sleep starts. Woken up violently due to lack of oxygen, often with tingling or numbness in limbs

An example of the influences of some of my cofactor deficiencies on cardiorespiratory symptoms:

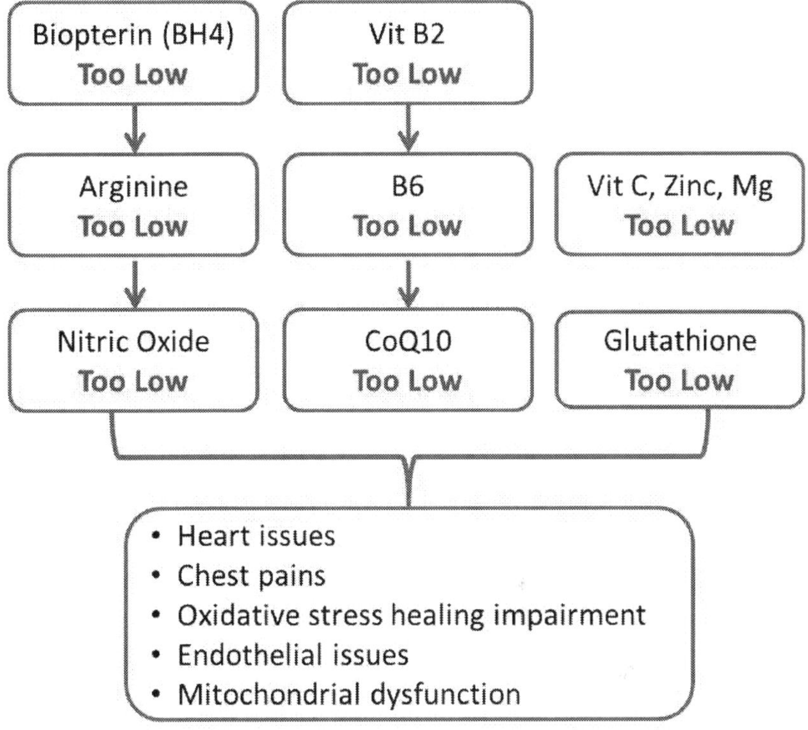

6. Musculoskeletal Symptoms

Musculoskeletal Issues 1

- Paresthesia: mostly numbness, but also ants crawling, electrical zaps, and burning sensations of hands, fingers, fingertips, feet, some toes, left knee, left arm, left ankle, elbows, lips, head
- Catabolic: breaking down tissue, muscle and bone for essential nutrients
- Rapid muscle weight loss
- Rapid bone density loss, osteopenia
- Left shoulder dropped
- Coordination issues, clumsiness, balance difficulties, walking difficulties
- Inability to pick up or hold cutlery due to strength, weakness and numbness
- Skin rash, bumps, crusty areas, small red spots that would spontaneously bleed

Musculoskeletal Issues 2

- Lots of cartilage crackling
- Joint inflammation that would not heal
- Endothelial: circulation impairment, swelling of fingertips by nail's matrix
- Odd itchy spells on nose, knees, legs, neck not satisfied by scratching
- Light scratching would cause red welts
- Burning eyelids sensation
- Eyesight issues: intermittent blurry vision, lack of focus, night blindness, many more floaters
- Unexplained bruises and easy bruising
- Hard to heal wounds, easy staph infections
- Oxidative stress showing on skin as liver spots
- Calcium plasma levels higher

Pains

- Lower- and mid-back
- Neck
- Joints
- Nerve
- Bone
- Shin
- Skin
- Chest
- Thigh muscles post sleep
- Chest muscles, pectoralis minor
- In between ribs
- Breastbone deep
- Shoulder blade
- Headaches
- Back seizing up completely
- Skin sunburn feeling without sun
- Cannot get comfortable
- Cannot find a good sleeping position

An example of the influences of some of my cofactor deficiencies on musculoskeletal symptoms:

Vitamin D **Too Low**	Magnesium **Too Low**
Amino Acids **Too Low**	Omega-3 **Too Low**
Testosterone **Too Low**	Vitamins B2, B6 **Too Low**
Vitamin K **Too Low**	Vitamins B9, B12 **Too Low**

7. ME/CFS Symptoms

There is an overlap of symptoms listed in the sections above and those that are often associated with Chronic Fatigue Syndrome (ME/CFS), because some are closely linked. There are many potential causes of CFS, but in my case it was due to exocrine pancreatic insufficiency (EPI) causing extensive nutrient deficiencies. This in turn caused the secondary (i.e., not by birth) mitochondrial dysfunction, and metabolism issues. There is a very helpful book I have listed in the Appendix which explains CFS and the mitochondrial dysfunction link in detail.

Mitochondria are essential organelles in animal and plant cells which are, simply put, the energy power plants of our cells. ATP (adenosine triphosphate) is the energy storage that they produce. They are in almost all our cells, and the heart, liver, pancreas, kidneys and muscles contain large amounts due to their high energy demand. Any dysfunction in the mitochondria can have a large impact on your health.

It is tough when you can barely get out of bed or almost faint when you sit or stand up. There were many days where I could barely move and felt like my body was shutting down and in survival mode. For weeks it was too hard to even talk, as I did not have enough spare breath or energy. Having enough energy to take a shower standing up or walking down the stairs was a milestone. Your heart and brain functions deteriorate drastically, and can cause heart arrhythmias, blood pressure swings, weakness, memory loss, confusion, brain fog, stuttering, dyslexia, etc. It is difficult to absorb information that is coming to you either from someone talking to you or from the TV. Some days I could not remember the names of my immediate family members or simple words used in everyday life. Since the pancreas requires a lot of healthy functioning mitochondria, this organ is also affected, causing a vicious cycle that hampers healing further.

You cannot function properly or at all with CFS, and it is a painful message from your body to force you to stop, rest and heal. Sometimes you cannot visibly see if someone has CFS, which often makes it even more painful and difficult to get the medical attention you need. How often are people suffering from CFS told it is in their head? Sad!

But without tackling the primary cause(s), which in my case was EPI, CFS will not be resolved, and can linger for many miserable years. Even during the healing period, the available energy level can swing wildly between days, and even intra-day. One minute you feel ready to go outside for a short walk, and the next minute you are curled in a ball and back in your bed. Pacing yourself during this period is difficult, but overdoing things will set you back considerably.

The list of CFS symptoms is massive, and these are just a few commonly mentioned ones I had:

Chronic Fatigue Syndrome (ME/CFS)

- Constant fatigue and malaise
- No energy and no stamina
- No concentration, brain fog, confusion
- Neurological issues, added sensitivities
- Motor impairments, weakness
- Dizziness and faintness
- Body ache and flu-like symptoms
- Post exertional fatigue and malaise (PEM)
- Heart rhythm issues
- Gastrointestinal issues
- Breathing, oxygen absorption issues
- ATP generation issues

8. Blood Tests Symptoms

#	Blood Tests	Notes
1	Insulin	As high as 17 μU/ml. Healthy is <3.
2	Glucose	As high as 120 mg/dL fasted with random checks over 250 mg/dL. Healthy fasted is <100. During hypoglycemia as low as 65 mg/dL.
3	Hemoglobin A1c (HbA1c)	As high as 5.9%. Healthy is <5.3.
4	Triglycerides	As high as 225 mg/dL. Healthy is <100. High triglycerides levels also cause higher LDL levels.
5	Triglycerides-to-HDL ratio	As high as 5.5. Healthy is <2.
6	HDL (high-density lipoprotein) cholesterol	As low as 30 mg/dL. Healthy is 60-90 mg/dL.
7	Total cholesterol-to-HDL ratio	As high as 5.9. Healthy is <3.5.
8	LDL (low-density lipoprotein) cholesterol	As high as 146. Healthy is <130.
9	Adiponectin	As low as 6 μg/mL. Healthy is >14.
10	Apo B (Apolipoprotein B-100)	As high as 107 mg/dL. Healthy is <60.
11	LDL-P	As high as 1744 nmol/L. Healthy is <1020. Insulin resistance, infections, metabolic syndrome are potential causes.
12	Candida IgA	High. Exposure to Candida yeast in the blood.

#	Blood Tests	Notes
13	Serotonin	Low normal. Can indicate deficiencies in tryptophan, L-carnitine and cofactors like vitamins B6, B9, C, zinc, copper, and magnesium.
14	Dopamine	High. Along with high norepinephrine can indicate deficiencies in copper and vitamin B6 due to issues with conversion.
15	Tiglylglycine (TG)	Slightly elevated. Can point to mitochondrial, energy production disorders, fatty acid beta-oxidation, autism, Parkinson's, cancer.
16	Cadmium , lead, mercury	Low but measurable when not provoked by chelation.
17	Calcium	High normal at 10 mg/dL. Corrected for albumin as high as 10.8 mg/dL. Can be tied to low vitamin K (needed to bind with calcium), or high vitamin D supplementation, which helps increase absorption of calcium from food. High levels can cause bone pain, muscle weakness and depression.
18	Osteocalcin	Low-normal. Helps take calcium from blood circulation and bind it to bone matrix, which requires vitamin K.
19	Vitamin K2	Deficient.
20	Vitamin D	Insufficient. As low as 25.7 ng/mL. Healthy is around 40-50.
21	Omega-3 Index	Low.

#	Blood Tests	Notes
22	Copper	Insufficient. Copper-to-zinc ratio of 0.7-1.0 is important. Mine was as low as 0.5. A cofactor in metabolic pathways involved in energy production, protection of cells from free radical damage, strengthening connective tissue, brain neurotransmitter function, iron absorption, storage and metabolism. Excess zinc-to-copper intake can cause copper deficiency.
23	Zinc	Insufficient. Copper-to-zinc ratio of 0.7-1.0 is important. Mine was as low as 0.5. Impacts immunity, protein metabolism, heme synthesis, growth, reproduction, digestion, wound healing and antioxidant function. Deficiency can be caused by malabsorption, alcoholism, chronic diarrhea, diabetes, excess copper or iron, diuretics, ACE inhibitors, or H2 blockers.
24	Potassium	Low. Indicates poor dietary intake, malabsorption, diarrhea, disease or certain medications. Can cause difficulty neutralizing acids from proteins. It helps maintain proper pH and normal water balance between the cells and body fluids. Muscle contractions, nerve impulses and blood pressure rely on availability of potassium. Licorice can cause low potassium levels and high blood pressure due to Glycyrrhizic acid.
25	Iron	As low as 55 μg/dL.

#	Blood Tests	Notes
26	Ratio of total testosterone-to-estradiol	As low as 7. Healthy is 30-40 for a male in his 40s.
27	Testosterone	As low as 349 ng/dL. Average is close to 600 for a male around 40.
28	Free Testosterone	As low at 0.69 ng/dL. At 2% of average, this should be around 12 ng/dL for a 40 year old male.
29	Ratio of free-to-total testosterone	As low as 0.2%. Healthy is ~2%.
30	Estradiol	As high as 87.5 pg/mL.
31	Alkaline phosphatase (ALP)	As low as 35 IU/L. Can indicate malnutrition, protein, zinc, folic acid, phosphorous, vitamins B6, and C deficiencies. High ALP can sometimes point to a vitamin D deficiency.
32	Aspartate aminotransferase (AST)	Low normal at 12 IU/L. Can indicate vitamin B6 deficiency.
33	Homocysteine	As high as 10.8 μmol/L. Healthy is 7-9. Linked to vitamin B9 and B12 deficiencies. Marker of potential cardiovascular issues. MTHFR C677T and A1298C mutations can cause lower production of L-methyl folate and hinder the synthesis of homocysteine to methionine and SAM-e. Betaine can help lower it.
34	Norepinephrine	Low. Along with high dopamine can indicate deficiencies in copper and vitamin B6.

9. Stool Tests Symptoms

#	Stool Tests	Notes
35	Fecal lipids 24 hour	High at 13 grams. Double normal levels on a low fat diet. <7 g on an expected 100 gram fat for the 24 hour test is normal.
36	Pancreatic Elastase	As low 38 as µg/mL. Healthy is > 200.
37	Dysbiotic flora	Too high levels of Morganella morganii, Alpha hemolytic strep, Gamma hemolytic strep, Kiebsiella pneumonia ssp pneumonia, Staphylococcus aureus, Pseudomonas aeruginosa. Missing beneficial bacteria Enterococcus spp.
38	Secretory IgA	Too low at 49.3 mg/dL. Indication of mucosal tissue levels, which acts as an immune barrier.
39	Total Short Chain Fatty Acids (SCFA)	High at 20 mg/mL.
40	Microscopic yeast	Too high.

10. Urine Tests Symptoms

#	Urine Tests	Notes
41	Cortisol	Low normal in the afternoon.
42	Cortisone	High normal over a 24 hour period.
43	DHEAS	Low normal.
44	a-Tetrahydro-cortisol (a-THF)	Too high.
45	Melatonin	Low normal. Could indicate low serotonin and thus low tryptophan amino acid, vitamins B6, B9, B12, magnesium, zinc or copper.
46	Kryptopyrrole (a.k.a. Mauve, Pyrrole, HPL)	Elevated at 434 µg/24hr. Oxidative stress marker and indication of vitamin B6 and zinc deficiencies as pyrroles bind to them. Also copper and manganese need to be watched.
Toxic Compounds		
47	2-Hydroxyiso-butyric Acid	Slightly elevated. Potential causes are MTBE/ETBE exposure, gasoline fumes, and water contamination. Methyl tert-butyl ether (MTBE) is a common gasoline additive. Consuming it through contaminated water may cause gastrointestinal irritation, liver and kidney damage, and nervous system effects.
48	Arsenic, cesium, cadmium, nickel, tungsten, tin, mercury, gadolinium.	Low but measurable toxic metals, when provoked by a DMSA chelator.

#	Urine Tests	Notes
49	Lead	Exceeds 3 times upper limit at 6.8 μg/g creatinine when provoked by DMSA chelator.
50	Thallium	Borderline high at 0.5 μg/g creatinine when provoked by DMSA chelator. Unprovoked was 0.4 μg/g creatinine. This can impact mitochondria and ATP generation, parathyroid, or heart rhythm issues. It replaces nutrient minerals such as potassium in enzymes functions. It is used as a gasoline additive, found in pesticides and electronics, but can also be on kale from thallium in soil. Potassium can help.
51	Phenylglyoxylic Acid	Elevated. Potential causes include styrene (Potential human carcinogen) exposure from, e.g., to-go cups, restaurant food containers, and commercial products like rubber, plastic, insulation, fiberglass, pipes, and carpet backing.
52	Thiodiglycolic Acid	Elevated. Potential causes are vinyl chloride, PVC exposure, lots of onions, B12 administration or stimulation of sulfur amino acid. It is used in shower curtains, car plastics, cling wrap, inflatable toys, mattresses, and flooring.

11. Nutrition Organic Acid Tests Symptoms

Please note that this section is a large reference table spanning dozens of pages since these tests are so comprehensive. It is a great example of biochemistry in practice and contains a lot of background information on metabolite test markers. Jump forward to Chapter 3 if you would like to skip the table at this point.

#	Test Marker	Note
53	**Type**: Urine **Area:** Methylation **Marker**: Methylation pathway	Imbalances found. Enzymatic process critical for DNA, estrogen and neurotransmitter metabolism, detoxification, immune function, and energy production. B vitamins, methionine, magnesium, selenium are needed for thc cnzyme catechol-O-methyltransferase (COMT). It also impacts homocysteine.
54	**Type**: Urine **Area**: Malabsorption **Marker**: Nitrogen Insufficiency	Imbalances found. Indication of malabsorption and malnutrition through lack of protein digestion and absorption.
55	**Type**: Urine **Area**: Malabsorption **Marker**: Need for Pancreatic Enzymes	Imbalances found. Fat and protein maldigestion and malabsorption are shown by various low amino acid values. Can indicate exocrine pancreatic insufficiency (EPI), celiac disease, small intestine villous atrophy, small bowel bacterial overgrowth, or impaired digestive capacity.

56	**Type**: Urine **Area**: Malabsorption **Marker**: Phenylacetic Acid	High. Can indicate intestinal bacterial dysbiosis. A by-product of Clostridia. Can indicate gastric hypochlorhydria or pepsin inactivity, impaired digestive peptidase function in the small intestine, insufficient absorption or mucosal transport in the small intestine, abnormal intestinal motility (partly regulated by cholecystokinin and secretin), or presence of colonic or other bacteria in the small intestine. If the essential amino acid phenylalanine is not sufficiently digested and absorbed in the small intestine, it is carried to the large bowel where anaerobic bacteria convert it to phenylethylamine. Can point to low BH4.
57	**Type**: Urine **Area**: Bacterial Dysbiosis **Marker**: Dihydroxy-phenylpropionic Acid (DHPPA)	High. Can indicate increased amounts of E. coli, Lactobacilli or Bifidobacteria.
58	**Type**: Urine **Area**: Bacterial Dysbiosis **Marker**: 3-Hydroxyphenylacetic Acid	High. Can indicate intestinal dysbiosis.
59	**Type**: Urine **Area**: Bacterial Dysbiosis **Marker**: 4-Hydroxyhippuric	High. Can indicate bacterial overgrowth, or excessive intake of fruits such as blueberries, or exposure to parabens (in, e.g., food additives, cosmetics) which have an estrogenic impact.

60	**Type**: Urine **Area**: Bacterial Dysbiosis **Marker**: 3,4 dihydroxy-phenylpropionic acid (34DHPPA)	High. Beneficial bacteria such as Lactobacilli, Bifido, E. Coli, but also dysbiotic bacteria Clostridia Orbiscindens break down chlorogenic acid into 34DHPPA. Can also indicate excessive intake of chlorogenic acid common in fruits, vegetables and juices.
61	**Type**: Urine **Area**: Bacterial Dysbiosis **Marker**: HPHPA	Elevated. By-product of Clostridia bacteria. It can inhibit metabolism of dopamine to epinephrine and norepinephrine.
62	**Type**: Urine **Area**: Bacterial Dysbiosis **Marker**: Benzoic Acid	High. Can indicate intestinal dysbiosis of gut microflora or metabolism of phenylalanine and dietary polyphenols. Can also point to high intake of berries, cranberries, food additive, preservative, polyphenols or phenylalanine.
63	**Type**: Urine **Area**: Bacterial Dysbiosis **Marker**: Hippuric Acid	High. Can point to intestinal dysbiosis. Benzoic acid is a by-product of gut bacteria and is also used as a food and beverage preservative. Can also be caused by chemical solvent exposure toluene (from out-gassing of building materials, carpets, glues). The liver combines benzoic acid and glycine to form hippuric acid.
64	**Type**: Urine **Area**: Yeast/ Fungal Dysbiosis **Marker**: Citramalic Acid	High. Produced mainly by Saccharomyces fungus species or Propionibacteria overgrowth
65	**Type**: Urine **Area**: Yeast/Fungal Dysbiosis **Marker**: Tricarballylic	High. Inhibits the Krebs cycle. By-product from Fumonisins fungal toxins. Elevated levels can be caused by corn-based food intake contaminated with fumonisins.

66	**Type**: Urine **Area**: Yeast/ Fungal Dysbiosis **Marker**: Furan-2,5-dicarboxylic	High. Indicates yeast/fungal overgrowth in the GI tract as it is a by-product of Aspergillus fungus.
67	**Type**: Urine **Area**: Yeast/Fungal Dysbiosis **Marker**: Arabinose	High. Indicates yeast/fungal overgrowth in GI tract as it is a by-product of Candida yeast. It is also a sugar in apples, grapes, and pears.
68	**Type**: Urine **Area**: Mitochondrial & Cell Energy **Marker**: Lactic Acid	No issue when low. It is a by-product of glycolysis, the anaerobic (i.e., not requiring oxygen) metabolic pathway which is the less efficient ATP production cycle. Oxidative phosphorylation (OxPhos) is the more efficient aerobic (i.e., using oxygen) metabolic pathway for ATP production. When elevated it can also indicate bacterial overgrowth in the GI tract, mitochondrial dysfunction, or vigorous exercise.
69	**Type**: Urine **Area**: Mitochondrial & Cell Energy **Marker**: Mitochondrial Dysfunction	Imbalances found. Mitochondria generate reactive oxygen species. Oxidative damage is considered an important factor in decline of physiologic function that occurs with aging and stress. Mitochondrial defects have been identified in cardiovascular disease, fatigue syndromes, neurologic disorders such as Parkinson's and Alzheimer's disease, as well as a variety of genetic conditions. Common nutritional deficiencies can impair mitochondrial efficiency.

70	**Type**: Urine **Area**: Mitochondrial & Cell Energy **Marker**: β-OH-Butyric Acid (BHBA)	High. It is a ketone formed from acetyl CoA and indicates ketosis from carbohydrate unavailability (e.g., fasting, diabetes strenuous exercise, ketogenic diet)
71	**Type**: Urine **Area**: Mitochondrial & Cell Energy **Marker**: 3-MethylGlutaric	Elevated. Reduced capacity to metabolize amino acid leucine can indicate mitochondrial dysfunction. Consider vitamins B2, B7, E, CoQ10, L-carnitine, acetyl-L-carnitine, and nicotinamide supplementation.
72	**Type**: Urine **Area**: Mitochondrial & Cell Energy **Marker**: 3-HydroxyGlutaric	Elevated. Reduced capacity to metabolize lysine and tryptophan and can indicate mitochondrial dysfunction or L-carnitine deficiency.
73	**Type**: Urine **Area**: Mitochondrial & Cell Energy **Marker**: 3-MethylGlutaconic	Elevated. Reduced capacity to metabolize amino acid leucine can indicate mitochondrial dysfunction. Consider vitamins B2, B7, E, CoQ10, L-carnitine, acetyl-L-carnitine, and nicotinamide supplementation.
74	**Type**: Urine **Area**: Mitochondrial & Cell Energy **Marker**: Pyruvic	High. Indicates impaired metabolism due to vitamins B1, B2, B3, B5, magnesium, lipoic acid cofactor insufficiencies or toxic metals (Arsenic, lead, mercury, and cadmium) exposure, muscle injury, severe adrenal insufficiency, or impaired conversion of pyruvate to alanine.

75	**Type**: Urine **Area**: Mitochondrial & Cell Energy **Marker**: Cis-Aconitic Acid	Low. Can point to low glutathione due to oxidative stress, which can inhibit the aconitase enzyme through toxic elements mercury, arsenic, antimony, fluoride (added to tap water). This enzyme requires cysteine, glutathione and ferrous iron so it could point to deficiencies. If precursor citric acid is not low as well it may indicate low carbohydrate diets, fasting or anorexic conditions. With normal or elevated citric acid and low cis-aconitic acid, it may be the result of urinary citrate wasting (leading to deficiencies) or of weakness in the enzyme that transforms citrate into cis-aconitate.
76	**Type**: Urine **Area**: Mitochondrial & Cell Energy **Marker**: Isocitric Acid	High. Can indicate vitamins B3, B12, magnesium, or manganese deficiencies.
77	**Type**: Urine **Area**: Mitochondrial & Cell Energy **Marker**: Fumaric	High. Points to impaired Krebs cycle, a defect in the mitochondrial function or enzyme fumarase.
78	**Type**: Urine **Area**: Mitochondrial & Cell Energy **Marker**: Succinic Acid	Low. Not burning amino acids as fuel at a normal rate. Can point to low vitamins B2, B6, B7, B9, B12, CoQ10 and thus BH4. It donates electrons to the mitochondrial electron transport and leads to formation of fumaric acid. Can be linked with lacto-ovo vegetarian diets, malabsorption and chronic fatigue.

79	**Type**: Urine **Area**: Mitochondrial & Cell Energy **Marker**: Malic Acid	High. Can indicate vitamins B2, B3 deficiency or yeast overgrowth.
80	**Type**: Urine **Area**: Mitochondrial & Cell Energy **Marker**: 2-Oxoglutaric	High. Can be due to dietary insufficiencies of vitamins B1, B2, B5, and Lipoic Acid.
81	**Type**: Urine **Area**: Mitochondrial & Cell Energy **Marker**: Aconitic	Low. If high could indicate mitochondrial disorders, deficiency in glutathione. Aconitase, the enzyme that metabolizes citric and aconitic acids, is dependent upon glutathione.
82	**Type**: Urine **Area**: Mitochondrial & Cell Energy **Marker**: Citric	High. Can indicate impaired metabolism due to toxic metals (e.g., mercury, arsenic), high yeast in the intestines, depletion of glutathione, high intake of citric acid, or metabolic acidosis.
83	**Type**: Urine **Area**: Neurotransmitter **Marker**: Vanylmandelic (VMA)	Slightly low. Can indicate lower production of neurotransmitter norepinephrine or epinephrine (adrenaline). It could be Clostridia bacteria inhibiting conversion from dopamine or low phenylalanine, tyrosine, magnesium, vitamin B6, or biopterin (BH4) levels.

84	**Type**: Urine **Area**: Neurotransmitter **Marker**: Homovanillic (HVA)	High. It is a metabolite of dopamine. Points to lowered conversion of dopamine to norepinephrine and epinephrine. Stress induced catecholamine output from the adrenal gland depletes vitamin C. This could indicate deficiencies in vitamin C or copper. Or caused by toxic metal exposure (e.g., lead, mercury, aluminium), intake of L-DOPA, dopamine, phenylalanine, or tyrosine supplements, catecholamine-secreting tumors, Clostridia bacteria or toxoplasmosis infection. If HVA is low, it could point to catecholamine metabolism or deficiency of dopamine beta-hydrolase perhaps due to low vitamin B6, magnesium, biopterin (BH4), phenylalanine or tyrosine.
85	**Type**: Urine **Area**: Neurotransmitter **Marker**: Vanilmandelic Acid (VMA)	Low. If VMA is low relative to HVA it can indicate low copper or low vitamin C. Low vitamin C would be consistent with low glutathione, because glutathione recycles vitamin C. It is a metabolite of norepinephrine and epinephrine, and low levels can indicate low production of those neurotransmitters, or deficient intake of tyrosine or phenylalanine, vitamin B6, magnesium or biopterin (BH4). It also can be caused by enzyme blockage of conversion of dopamine to norepinephrine by Clostridia bacteria byproducts.

86	**Type**: Urine **Area**: Neurotransmitter **Marker**: HVA/VMA ratio	High. Shows a lowered conversion of dopamine to norepinephrine and epinephrine. Could indicate deficiency in vitamin C or copper, Clostridia bacteria overgrowth as this inhibits the enzyme, toxic metal exposure, intake of L-DOPA, dopamine, phenylalanine, tyrosine, catecholamine-secreting tumors, or toxoplasmosis infection.
87	**Type**: Urine **Area**: Neurotransmitter **Marker**: 3-Methyl-4-OH-phenylglycol	Low. It is a metabolite of norepinephrine degradation. Can indicate low precursors phenylalanine, dopamine, noradrenalin, or low cofactor vitamins B2, B3, B6, magnesium, or iron. Or can indicate impaired methylation if VMA is also low.
88	**Type**: Urine **Area**: Neurotransmitter **Marker**: Kynurenic Acid	Low. Can indicate low vitamins B2, B3, B6, high tryptophan supplementation, chronic infections, or low picolinic acid.
89	**Type**: Urine **Area**: Nutritional **Marker**: a-Ketoadipic acid	High. Made from tryptophan and lysine via alpha-aminoadipic acid and is a precursor of glutaric acid. It also is a by-product of yeast. Could indicate yeast overgrowth. Could also be due to high glutaric acid, impaired metabolism due to cofactor vitamins B1, B2, B3, B5, magnesium, cysteine, or lipoic acid insufficiencies, or toxic metal exposure (Arsenic, mercury, antimony, cadmium). It is also linked to biopterin (BH4).

90	**Type**: Urine **Area**: Neurotransmitter **Marker**: 5-Hydroxy-indoleacetio or 5-OH-indoleacetic Acid (5-HIAA)	Low. It is a breakdown product from tryptophan and can indicate low serotonin production and be a cause of depression. Inflammation uses serotonin with the MAO-A enzyme. If high it can point to increased release of serotonin from gut or use of SSRIs.
91	**Type**: Urine **Area**: Neurotransmitter **Marker**: Quinolinic	High. Can indicate chronic inflammation from microbial infections, central nervous system degeneration, excessive tryptophan supplementation, or exposure to environmental phthalates (used in plastics).
92	**Type**: Urine **Area**: Neurotransmitter **Marker**: Quinolinic / 5-HIAA ratio	High. Can point to neural excitotoxicity, excessive inflammation, recurrent infections, excess cortisol due to stress, or high exposure to phthalates in plastics. Quinolinic acid is derived from amino acid tryptophan, which makes the cofactor nicotinamide adenine dinucleotide (NAD). Carnitine, melatonin, capsaicin, turmeric (contains curcumin) and garlic may reduce brain damage from high Quinolinic. Niacin or niacinamide may reduce quinolinic acid by decreasing tryptophan shunting. 5-HTP supplementation can help for low 5-HIAA.
93	**Type**: Urine **Area**: Neurotransmitter **Marker**: Homogentisic Acid	High. Can indicate impaired metabolism due to cofactor insufficiency iron or vitamin C. Rarely is it tied to a genetic disorder homogentisic aciduria.

94	**Type**: Urine **Area**: Bacterial Dysbiosis **Marker**: 2-Hydroxy-phenylacetic Acid	High. Can indicate bacterial dysbiosis, perhaps Proteus bacteria. Can also indicate excessive phenylalanine or tyrosine, reduced oxygenation, iron deficiency, anemia, pulmonary disorder. Can indicate low vitamins C, B9, or BH4.
95	**Type**: Urine **Area**: Nutritional **Marker**: Need for Probiotics	Intestinal dysbiosis found. Probiotics can help with production of some B and K vitamins, enhance digestion and absorption, immune function and intestinal permeability. Alterations of gastrointestinal microflora may result from C-section delivery, antibiotic use, cleaning products, chlorine and ammonia in tap water, certain herbicides, decreased consumption of fermented foods and use of certain drugs. Some of the diseases associated with microflora imbalances include IBS, IBD, fibromyalgia, Chronic Fatigue Syndrome, obesity, atopic illness, colic and cancer.
96	**Type**: Urine **Area**: Nutritional **Marker**: Vitamin A	Insufficient. It is fat-soluble. It impacts vision, antioxidant and immune function, gene expression and cell growth. Can be linked to chronic alcoholism, zinc deficiency, hypothyroidism, and oral contraceptives.
97	**Type**: Urine **Area**: Nutritional **Marker**: B1 - Thiamin	Insufficient. Impacts energy production from food, synthesis of ATP, DNA, RNA and NADPH. Deficiency can cause neuropathy, muscle weakness, cardiac problems, edema, encephalopathy, or dementia.

98	**Type**: Urine **Area**: Nutritional **Marker**: B2 - Riboflavin	Insufficient. Impacts antioxidant function, energy production, detoxification, methionine metabolism and vitamin activation (e.g., B6). Deficiency can cause oxidative stress, mitochondrial dysfunction, low uric acid, low vitamins B3 or B6, high homocysteine, anemia, or throat inflammation.
99	**Type**: Urine **Area**: Nutritional **Marker**: B3 - Niacin	Insufficient. Impacts NAD and NADP, energy production from food, fatty acid and cholesterol synthesis, cell signaling, DNA repair and cell differentiation. It can be caused by deficiencies in tryptophan, vitamins B6, B2 or iron. Deficiency can cause, e.g., dermatitis, diarrhea, dementia, depression, memory loss, or fatigue.
100	**Type**: Urine **Area**: Nutritional **Marker**: B6 - Pyridoxine	Insufficient. Can be due to malabsorption or dysbiosis. Impacts glycogenolysis, gluconeogenesis, neurotransmitters, heme, vitamin B3, red blood cells, and nucleic acids. Deficiency can cause irritability, depression, seizures, oral inflammation, impaired immunity or increased homocysteine.
101	**Type**: Urine **Area**: Nutritional **Marker**: B9 - Folic Acid	Insufficient. Impacts DNA and SAMe, methylation, nucleic acids, amino acid metabolism, red blood cells. Can be caused by high-dose NSAIDs, diabetic medicine, H2 blockers, diuretics, anti-convulsants, or SSRIs. Deficiency can cause anemia, fatigue, low methionine, higher homocysteine, impaired immunity, or heart disease.

102	**Type**: Urine **Area**: Nutritional **Marker**: B12 - Cobalamin	Insufficient. Impacts energy production from fats and proteins, methylation, hemoglobin, red blood cells, nerve cells, DNA and RNA. Can be caused by malabsorption, hypochlorhydria, gastritis, H. pylori, H2 blockers, PPIs, vegan diets, diabetic medicine. Can cause anemia, fatigue, paresthesia, memory loss, depression, dementia, methylation defects, or chromosome breaks.
103	**Type**: Urine **Area**: Nutritional **Marker**: Vitamin C - Ascorbic Acid	Low. Antioxidant. Impacts cholesterol, white blood cells, antibodies, collagen, glutathione, norepinephrine and carnitine. Deficiency can be caused by contraceptives, aspirin, diuretics, NSAIDs, or malabsorption.
104	**Type**: Urine **Area**: Nutritional **Marker**: Vitamin E	Insufficient. Antioxidant, fat-soluble. It impacts cell signaling, immune function, and coagulation. Deficiency may occur with malabsorption and certain drugs. Can cause peripheral neuropathy, ataxia, muscle weakness, retinopathy, and increased risk of CVD, prostate cancer and cataracts.
105	**Type**: Urine **Area**: Nutritional **Marker**: Cystathionine	Low. Made from methionine. Can indicate low glutathione, vitamins B6, B9, B12, cysteine or serine. Cystathionine is preceded by homocysteine. Cystathionine formation from homocysteine requires serine and vitamin B6
106	**Type**: Urine **Area**: Nutritional **Marker**: Alpha-amino-N-Butyrate	Low. Indication of vitamins B6, B9, or B12 insufficiencies.

107	**Type**: Urine **Area**: Nutritional **Marker**: 3-Methylhistidine	High. Burning protein at a higher rate than average. This can mean deficiencies in vitamins B2, B6, B9, and B12. It is derived from skeletal muscle and indicates abnormal catabolism of muscle or a degenerative condition. High levels suggest increased uptake of short-chain peptides, possibly increased gut permeability, and increased hydrolysis of short-chain dietary peptides in blood, liver and spleen. Tied to high threonine
108	**Type**: Urine **Area**: Nutritional **Marker**: Formimino-glutamic Acid	High. Produced from histidine. Can indicate vitamins B6, B9, or B12 deficiency due to, e.g., malabsorption, impaired folate metabolism, severe oxidative stress, excessive histidine supplementation, or a partial block in methionine synthase. Consistent with glutathione depletion. Can also indicate impaired methylation, high homocysteine, "methyl trap" due to low B12 (compromised recycling of tetrahydrofolate). It can also be tied to rare disorders in purine synthesis, homocystinuria and a predisposition to cardiovascular disease.
109	**Type**: Urine **Area**: Nutritional **Marker**: Isovalerylglycine	High. Indicates insufficiencies in vitamins B2, B7, carnitine, or CoQ10.
110	**Type**: Urine **Area**: Nutritional **Marker**: Xanthurenic Acid	High. It is a metabolite of tryptophan. Can indicate high estrogen, vitamin B6 deficiency, or excess tryptophan intake.

111	**Type**: Urine **Area**: Nutritional **Marker**: 3-Hydroxy-propionic acid	Low. Glutamate metabolite of propionic acid, a precursor of methylmalonic acid. If high can indicate vitamins B7, B12 and magnesium insufficiencies.
112	**Type**: Urine and blood **Area**: Nutritional **Marker**: Magnesium	Insufficient. Impacts >300 metabolic reactions, e.g., ATP energy production, bone formation, muscle and nerve conduction, cell signaling. Deficiency can be caused by malabsorption, alcoholism, hyperparathyroidism, renal disorders, diabetes, diuretics, or high zinc. Can cause muscle weakness, tremors, spasms, constipation, fatigue, depression, hypertension, arrhythmias, hypocalcemia, personality changes, or inhibit antioxidant functions.
113	**Type**: Urine **Area**: Nutritional **Marker**: Methylmalonic	Elevated. Indicates vitamin B12 deficiency.
114	**Type**: Urine **Area**: Nutritional **Marker**: Methylcitric	Elevation usually indicates a biotin (vitamin H) deficiency, which may be due to malabsorption, excessive intake of raw egg white, dietary deficiency or dysbiosis.
115	**Type**: Urine **Area**: Nutritional **Marker**: Phosphoric	Low. Can indicate (pseudo) hypoparathyroidism, low intake, or a vitamin D deficiency. Phosphorus is important for bones, acid-base balance, DNA, ATP, and phospholipids. Deficiency can cause bone pain.

116	**Type**: Urine **Area**: Nutritional **Marker**: 3-Hydroxy-3-Methylglutaric	High. Indicates deficiency in CoQ10.
117	**Type**: Urine **Area**: Nutritional **Marker**: Molybdenum	Insufficient. Impacts conversion of sulfites to sulfate, and nucleotides to uric acid. It helps metabolize aldehydes, other toxins and breaks down acetaldehyde, which along with ethanol, is a by-product of Candida. May be caused by increased sulfite, decreased plasma uric acid, decreased antioxidant function, deficient sulfate, impaired sulfation (detoxification), and neurologic disorders. Sulfite oxidase issues can impair dopamine and noradrenaline synthesis. Sulfites can inhibit lung and liver cell ATP energy production, deplete glutathione, or cause fatigue.
118	**Type**: Urine **Area**: Nutritional **Marker**: Glutaric Acid	High. Can point to deficiencies in vitamin B2, CoQ10, carnitine, or fatty acid oxidation impairment, glutaryl CoA metabolism impairment, malabsorption, intestinal dysbiosis, celiac, or too much medium-chain triglycerides (MCT oil) intake. Formed from lysine, tryptophan and vitamin B2.
119	**Type**: Urine **Area**: Nutritional **Marker**: N-AcetylCysteine	Low. Powerful antioxidant, glutathione precursor and chelating agent. If high, it is usually due to supplementation of NAC.
120	**Type**: Urine **Area**: Nutritional **Marker**: Pantothenic	High. High points to a high intake of vitamin B5. Low points to malabsorption and vitamin B5 deficiency.

121	**Type**: Urine **Area**: Nutritional **Marker**: Pyridoxic	Low. Can indicate vitamin B6 deficiency, defective absorption or intestinal dysbiosis.
122	**Type**: Urine **Area**: Toxin & Detoxification **Marker**: a-Ketophenylacetic acid	Elevated. Indicates exposure to styrene from, e.g., to-go food and beverage containers. Can cause glutathione depletion in the detoxification process.
123	**Type**: Urine **Area**: Toxin & Detoxification **Marker**: Pyroglutamic Acid	High. Points to intracellular glutathione deficiency due to, e.g., toxic exposure like acetaminophen toxicity, DDT, PCBs, halogenated carbons, certain antibiotics, genetic deficiency of glutathione synthetase, enzyme oxoprolinase. Can cause glycine deficiency, urea disorders, propionic acidemia, or homocystinuria.
124	**Type**: Urine **Area**: Toxin & Detoxification **Marker**: 2-Hydroxybutyric	High. Indicates glutathione deficiency. It is a ketone body produced as a by-product of fatty acids oxidation for energy.
125	**Type**: Urine **Area**: Toxin & Detoxification **Marker**: Orotic	High. If high points to excess ammonia.
126	**Type**: Urine **Area**: Toxin & Detoxification **Marker**: 2-Hydroxyhippuric	High. Can indicate high aspartame, salicylates, or intestinal bacterial overgrowth, which is converting tyrosine or phenylalanine to salicylic acid. 2-Hydroxyhippuric is a combination of salicylic acid and glycine.

127	**Type**: Blood, Urine **Area**: Amino Acids **Marker**: Arginine	Low. Can indicate vitamin B6 deficiency, protein malnutrition or maldigestion, poor diet or gastrointestinal dysfunction. It detoxifies ammonia, is a precursor of creatine and creatinine which are involved in muscle metabolism. Release of insulin by the pancreas is stimulated by arginine and transient hyper-, hypoglycemia can be a consequence of arginine deficiency. It is important to leukocytes and immune function and is documented to stimulate killer cell activity for phagocytosis. Low levels can cause muscle weakness, fatigue, impacted growth hormone, lack of cardio, and chronic infections.
128	**Type**: Blood **Area**: Amino Acids **Marker**: Histidine	Low. Required for tissue growth and copper transport. Indicates malnutrition or intestinal dysfunction. A precursor of histamine (vasodilator) which mediates some inflammatory responses and stimulates HCL gastric secretions for digestion of food. Deficient histidine can contribute to low stomach acid.
129	**Type**: Urine **Area**: Amino Acids **Marker**: Isoleucine	Low. Can indicate zinc deficiency, protein deficiency, gastrointestinal dysbiosis, malabsorption, or pancreatic insufficiency.
130	**Type**: Blood **Area**: Amino Acids **Marker**: Lysine	Low. Synthesis of other amino acids requires lysine along with vitamin B6. Some B6 deficiency symptoms are actually lysine deficiency limiting functional B6 activity.

131	**Type**: Urine **Area**: Amino Acids **Marker**: Leucine	Low. Indicates incomplete digestive proteolysis, leaky gut, pancreatic dysfunction, or zinc deficiency. It is the primary of 3 branched chain amino acids (BCAA) and an activator of the protein known as mTOR.
132	**Type**: Blood, Urine **Area**: Amino Acids **Marker**: Methionine	Low normal. Can indicate malabsorption, impaired methionine metabolism, methylation, trans-sulfuration, elevated homocysteine, low vitamins B6, B9, B12, serine, betaine, glycine, or magnesium
133	**Type**: Blood **Area**: Amino Acids **Marker**: Alanine	Low. Nonessential amino which can indicate protein gastrointestinal dysfunction, malnutrition or maldigestion. It may come directly from dietary protein, or it can be formed in body cells from serine or from pyruvic acid. Tryptophan and cysteine are minor sources of alanine. Sometimes adrenocortical insufficiency is caused by impaired conversion of pyruvic acid to alanine. It is a primary source of glucose with caloric insufficiency.
134	**Type**: Blood **Area**: Amino Acids **Marker**: Asparagine	Low. Indicates protein malnutrition or malabsorption. It can be synthesized from aspartate and glutamine.
135	**Type**: Blood **Area**: Amino Acids **Marker**: Aspartic Acid	Low. Synthesized from glutamate with vitamin B6. Indicates protein malnutrition or maldigestion and possible vitamin B6 deficiency. It is used in the biosynthesis of amino acids and is a precursor to methionine, threonine, isoleucine, and lysine. Used in the urea cycle and gluconeogenesis.

136	**Type**: Urine **Area**: Amino Acids **Marker**: Aspartate	Low. Synthesized from glutamate with vitamin B6. Indicates protein malnutrition or maldigestion and possible vitamin B6 deficiency. It is used in the biosynthesis of amino acids and is a precursor to methionine, threonine, isoleucine, and lysine. It is used in the urea cycle and gluconeogenesis.
137	**Type**: Urine **Area**: Amino Acids **Marker**: Citrulline	Low. Points to malabsorption, insufficient protein intake, or alcoholism. Can indicate magnesium deficiency, low ornithine, or limited ammonia detoxification.
138	**Type**: Blood **Area**: Amino Acids **Marker**: Cysteine	If low can indicate low vitamins B6 and B2, zinc, or magnesium for B6 synthesis. Can also indicate low glutathione as it is necessary (along with glycine and glutamine) in glutathione production.
139	**Type**: Blood **Area**: Amino Acids **Marker**: Cystine	Low. Cystine is the oxidized form of cysteine. In the form of cysteine it is a key component of glutathione, coenzyme A, many enzymes, and insulin. Low cystine points to protein malnutrition, gastrointestinal dysfunctions, impaired methionine metabolism, or oxidative stress.
140	**Type**: Blood **Area**: Amino Acids **Marker**: Glutamine	Low. Can indicate protein malnutrition, nitrogen imbalance, malabsorption, chronic alcoholism, or renal acidosis. It is a building block of glutathione. It can be made endogenously (in the body) by combining ammonia and glutamate.

141	**Type**: Urine **Area**: Amino Acids **Marker**: Phenylalanine	Low. Needed to produce tyrosine, neurotransmitters (dopamine, DOPA, epinephrine) and thyroid hormone. Low indicates protein malnutrition, malabsorption or low stomach acid (too high pH).
142	**Type**: Blood, Urine **Area**: Amino Acids **Marker**: Taurine	High. Can be due to excess intake or poor renal function. Taurine insufficiency can cause biliary insufficiency, fat malabsorption, cardiac arrhythmia, congestive heart failure, poor vision, retinal degeneration, immune dysfunction, enhanced inflammatory response to xenobiotics, convulsions and seizures. Deficient taurine may result in increased cellular calcium and sodium, reduced magnesium, or increased inflammatory response to toxins, foreign proteins, and chemicals. It is used in bile production, has neurotransmitter and antioxidant functions.
143	**Type**: Blood, Urine **Area**: Amino Acids **Marker**: Threonine	Low Can indicate malabsorption. Can cause high oxalates and B6, or B12 deficiencies.
144	**Type**: Blood, Urine **Area**: Amino Acids **Marker**: Tryptophan	Low. Required to produce niacin and serotonin. Indicates protein malnutrition, malabsorption or low stomach acid. Can impact BH4 and vitamins B3 or B6. If elevated it can be due to use of aspirin, acetylsalicylic acid or salicylates, which compete with tryptophan for binding to albumin.

145	**Type**: Blood **Area**: Amino Acids **Marker**: Proline	Low. Points to insufficient protein intake or malabsorption. Proline is a component of collagen and is metabolized from alpha-ketoglutarate, which in turn is a precursor of glutamate and glutamine, and is metabolic fuel for cells of the gastrointestinal tract. If proline is high it can point to poor collagen synthesis and insufficient vitamin C or niacin.
146	**Type**: Blood, Urine **Area**: Amino Acids **Marker**: Tyrosine	High. Can indicate the need for manganese, vitamin B6, or high intake of phenylalanine or tyrosine.
147	**Type**: Blood **Area**: Amino Acids **Marker**: Valine	High. Can indicate zinc, manganese, or vitamin B6 deficiencies. If low can indicate leaky gut or pancreatic dysfunction.
148	**Type**: Urine **Area**: Amino Acids **Marker**: 2-Hydroxyiso-valeric	Low. High can indicate vitamin B1 or lipoic acid deficiencies, lactic acidosis, or episodic ketosis. High levels have been linked with maple syrup urine disease, or pyruvate dehydrogenase deficiency.
149	**Type**: Urine **Area**: Amino Acids **Marker**: 2-Oxoisovaleric	Low. Elevations can indicate vitamin B1, lipoic acid, or pyruvate dehydrogenase deficiency.
150	**Type**: Urine **Area**: Amino Acids **Marker**: 2-Oxoisocaproic	Low. Elevations can indicate vitamin B1, lipoic acid, or pyruvate dehydrogenase deficiency.

151	**Type**: Urine **Area**: Amino Acids **Marker**: 2-Hydroxyiso-caproic	Low. Slight elevations can indicate vitamin B1 or lipoic acid deficiencies. High levels have been linked with maple syrup urine disease, short bowel syndrome, or pyruvate dehydrogenase deficiency.
152	**Type**: Urine **Area**: Amino Acids **Marker**: Mandelic	High. Usually caused by exposure to styrene (coffee cups, to-go containers). Can also be due to certain medications like antispasmodic or vasodilators, or phenylalanine supplements.
153	**Type**: Urine **Area**: Amino Acids **Marker**: Phenylpyruvic	Elevated. Can indicate intake of phenylalanine, deficiencies in B6, B9, or zinc, or issues with the production of biopterin, a cofactor required for phenylalanine metabolism.
154	**Type**: Urine **Area**: Amino Acids **Marker**: 4-Hydroxy-phenyllactic	Low. Slight increases may be due to increased tyrosine intake, bacterial gut metabolism, short bowel syndrome, or liver disease. High values can point to tyrosinemias, which can result from immature development of enzyme synthesis in infants or genetic deficiencies.
155	**Type**: Urine **Area**: Metabolites **Marker**: Uracil	Elevated. Indicates folic acid (B9) deficiency or a defect in folic acid metabolism. B9 is a methyl donor in conversion of uracil to thymine.
156	**Type**: Urine **Area**: Metabolites **Marker**: Thymine	Low. Indicates folic acid (B9) deficiency or a defect in folic acid metabolism. Vitamin B9 is a methyl donor in conversion of uracil to thymine.

157	**Type**: Urine **Area**: Metabolites **Marker**: Glyceric	Elevated. Can point to microbial sources such as yeast (Aspergillus, Penicillium, or Candida), or dietary sources of glycerol (glycerin).
158	**Type**: Urine **Area**: Metabolites **Marker**: Glycolic	Elevated. Oxalate metabolite. Can point to microbial sources such as yeast (Aspergillus, Penicillium, or Candida), dietary sources of glycerol (glycerin) or excessive fats if bile salt is deficient, unabsorbed fatty acids, fibromyalgia, malabsorption of fats, or anti-freeze exposure.
159	**Type**: Blood, Urine **Area**: Metabolites **Marker**: Phospho-Ethanolamine	Low. Can point to malabsorption, magnesium deficiency, protein insufficiency, or insufficient choline from dietary lecithin. Tied to vitamin B6 and SAMe. Can be made endogenously from serine via phosphorylation of ethanolamine. It is a precursor of phosphatidyl choline, choline and the neurotransmitter acetylcholine.
160	**Type**: Blood **Area**: Metabolites **Marker**: Glycine	Low. Used in the transsulfuration metabolic pathway as a step in the production of glutathione. It helps lower homocysteine, and is a methyl donor. Threonine and serine are important sources of glycine. After two days of fasting or in early stages of starvation, elevated glycine may occur from catabolism of body protein. Negative nitrogen balance and deficiencies of threonine and serine may accompany low glycine. Low glycine can also be due to detoxification of high benzoic acid (benzoate is a common food or drink preservative).

161	**Type**: Blood **Area**: Metabolites **Marker**: Ethanolamine	High. Can be because of high serine, or intestinal dysbiosis. If phosphoethanolamine is low relative to ethanolamine it suggests low intracellular magnesium.
162	**Type**: Blood **Area**: Metabolites **Marker**: Phosphoserine	Elevated. Can indicate magnesium or vitamin B6 deficiency causing incomplete synthesis to serine, or parathyroid dysfunction.
163	**Type**: Urine **Area**: Metabolites **Marker**: Oxalic	Elevated. Indicator of Candida, Aspergillus or Penicillum yeast, or bacteria overgrowth. Can also be due to high vitamin C, high intake of oxalate rich foods (e.g., spinach, raspberries, chocolate, wheat bran, peanuts) or exposure to pollutants. Malabsorption of fat, excessive fat in diet or deficient bile salts can also be a cause, since unabsorbed fatty acids bind with calcium, leaving less to bind with oxalic acid. High levels can contribute to kidney stones or reduced ionized calcium, reduced absorption of essential minerals like zinc, magnesium, and calcium. It can cause crystals to form in kidneys, joints, muscles, eyes, blood vessels, heart, etc. and could contribute to pain in fibromyalgia. Vitamins B6, E, chondroitin sulfate, taurine, selenium, omega-3, or arginine supplements can help reduce levels.

164	**Type**: Blood **Area**: Metabolites **Marker**: Serine	Elevated. Can indicate low vitamins B6, B9, manganese, betaine, hyperinsulinemia, or catabolism. It is required for the metabolism of fat, tissue growth and the immune system as it assists in the production of immunoglobulins and antibodies. It is interchangeable with glycine and used in the transsulfuration metabolic pathway as a step in the production of glutathione. It helps lower homocysteine, is a constituent of brain proteins and nerve sheaths. Low levels can indicate magnesium deficiency, methionine metabolism or acetylcholine synthesis issues.
165	**Type**: Blood **Area**: Metabolites **Marker**: Sarcosine	High. Metabolism requires B2 and could indicate vitamins B2 or B9 deficiencies.
166	**Type**: Blood **Area**: Dietary Peptide **Marker**: 1-Methylhistidine	High. Meat consumption marker. Derived mainly from the anserine (β-alanyl-L-1-methylhistidine) of dietary meat sources, especially fish or poultry. Can point to short-chain peptides, possibly increased gut permeability, and decreased activity of digestive peptidases in the small intestine.
167	**Type**: Blood **Area**: Dietary Peptide **Marker**: β-Alanine	Elevated. Meat consumption marker. Derived mainly from the anserine (β-alanyl-L-1-methylhistidine) of dietary meat sources, especially poultry, but can also be due to high fish oil.

168	**Type**: Blood **Area**: Oxidative Stress **Marker**: Glutathione	Low. Produced using cysteine, glutamine, glycine and cofactors vitamins C, E, B1, B2, B6, B9, B12, minerals selenium, magnesium and zinc, and alpha lipoic acid. It is a source of sulfate and key for antioxidant and detoxification activity. Use is increased with high-fat diets, cigarette smoke, cystinuria, chronic alcoholism, acetaminophen use, infection, inflammation and toxic exposure. Deficiency may result in oxidative stress and damage, impaired detoxification, altered immunity, macular degeneration and increased risk of chronic illness. This test combines both oxidized (bad) and reduced (good), but gives an indication.
169	**Type**: Blood **Area**: Oxidative Stress **Marker**: Coenzyme Q10 Ubiquinone	An antioxidant that is synthesized in the body and contained in cell membranes. It is essential for energy production and pH regulation. Deficiency can occur with statins, anti-diabetic medication or beta-blockers. Low levels may aggravate oxidative stress, diabetes, cancer, heart failure, arrhythmias, or neurologic diseases. My experience ties it to EPI as well, likely due to cofactor deficiencies.
170	**Type**: Urine **Area**: Oxidative Stress **Marker**: Lipid Peroxides	High. Reflects oxidative damage to polyunsaturated fatty acids, which are components of cell membranes.

171	**Type**: Blood **Area**: Fatty Acid Metabolism **Marker**: Eicosapen-taenoic (EPA Omega-3)	High due to too much fish oil supplements. This is usually low in Western diets. It is anti-inflammatory, and deficiencies lead to inflammation, arthritis, heart disease, and aging. Your body can produce limited amounts but requires sufficient ALA, zinc, magnesium, B3, B6, and C.
172	**Type**: Blood **Area**: Fatty Acid Metabolism **Marker**: Omega-3 %	High EPA or DHA indicates high fish oil consumption. It is fat from for example cold water fish, flax, or walnut.
173	**Type**: Blood **Area**: Fatty Acid Metabolism **Marker**: Eicosadienoic (Omega-6)	High. A product of gamma linolenic acid (GLA) and is used to produce dihomo-γ-Linolenic Acid (DGLA). High due to impaired conversion of GLA to DGLA (Delta - 6 desaturase Activity), which requires zinc.
174	**Type**: Blood **Area**: Fatty Acid Metabolism **Marker**: Arachidonic Acid (Omega-6)	Low. Possibly due to low DGLA, or Delta-5 desaturase not working well due to deficiencies in vitamins B2, B3, B6, C, insulin, zinc, or magnesium. It is a pro-inflammatory fatty acid and usually high due to corn oil, corn fed meat consumption. Synthesis is inhibited by NSAID drugs.
175	**Type**: Blood **Area**: Fatty Acid Metabolism **Marker**: Docosate-traenoic Acid (Omega-6)	Low. It is low since it is a product of DGLA, which showed in low levels.

176	**Type**: Blood **Area**: Fatty Acid Metabolism **Marker**: Dihomo-γ-Linolenic Acid DGLA (Omega-6)	Low. Due to diets low in both essential fatty acids, linoleic acid, or DGLA. It is anti-inflammatory. Insufficiency impairs cellular functions and tissue responses. Elongase reaction is not working well, and it points to deficiencies in vitamins B3, B5, B6, B7, or C. It can also point to high levels of saturated, monounsaturated, trans fatty acids, and slow cholesterol conversion of GLA to DGLA. An impaired conversion of GLA to DGLA (Delta - 6 desaturase enzyme activity) can be due to inadequate zinc, magnesium, or B3, B6, and C.
177	**Type**: Blood **Area**: Fatty Acid Metabolism **Marker**: Omega-6 %	Low. Fats from vegetable oil, grains, most meats, and dairy. It is usually too high with the modern Western diet.
178	**Type**: Blood **Area**: Fatty Acid Metabolism **Marker**: Oleic (Omega-9)	High. Points to too much olive oil intake. Helps maintain membrane fluidity, which is key for mitochondria and receptors in cells to function. Low levels can be improved with more olive oil consumption. It is usually too low with the modern Western diet.
179	**Type**: Blood **Area**: Fatty Acid Metabolism **Marker**: Vaccenic (Omega-7)	High due to too much olive oil intake. Monounsaturated fat, similar to oleic acid which helps maintain membrane fluidity, and is key for mitochondria and receptors in cells to function. Low levels can be improved with more olive oil. It is usually too low with the modern Western diet.

180	**Type**: Blood **Area**: Fatty Acid Metabolism **Marker**: Nervonic (Omega-9)	High. Due to high olive oil intake as my insulin levels are low. Usually low due to high carbohydrate diets that inhibit fatty acid synthesis. Insulinemia (high insulin) stimulates fatty acid synthesis and can cause high levels.
181	**Type**: Blood **Area**: Fatty Acid Metabolism **Marker**: Palmitic (Saturated)	Low. It is high in palm kernel and coconut oils. The liver can convert fatty acids into cholesterol of which palmitic acid is the most stimulatory. High levels can lead to increased serum cholesterol, increased risk of atherosclerosis, cardiovascular disease, and stroke.
182	**Type**: Blood **Area**: Fatty Acid Metabolism **Marker**: LA/DGLA Ratio	High/Impaired. Ratio of linoleic acid (LA) LA to dihomo-γ-linolenic (DGLA) increases when the delta 6 desaturase enzyme is inhibited by zinc and magnesium deficiency, elevated insulin, or dietary excess of saturated, monoenoic, or trans fatty acid.
183	**Type**: Blood **Area**: Fatty Acid Metabolism **Marker**: Stearic (Saturated)	High. Can indicate a high meat diet. Saturated fatty acid from meat, dairy, coconuts, or palm oils. Usually occurs with high serum triglycerides, which is a risk factor in atherosclerotic vascular disease.
184	**Type**: Blood **Area**: Fatty Acid Metabolism **Marker**: AA/EPA (Omega-6/Omega-3) Ratio	Low due to fish oil supplementation. Arachidonic acid (AA) and eicosapentaenoic acid (EPA) ratio. High ratio indicates an overabundance of the pro-inflammatory omega-6 fatty acid, quite common in Western high meat and corn oil diets. If the ratio is too high, taking omega-3 fatty acids, including EPA could help.

185	**Type**: Urine **Area**: Fatty Acid Metabolism **Marker**: 3-hydroxybutyric	High. Ketones, such as 3-hydroxybutyric and acetoacetic acids are the end-products of rapid or excessive fatty-acid breakdown. If elevated, points to prolonged fasting, protein malnutrition, high fat diet, vitamin B12 deficiency, severe GI Candida overgrowth, or pulmonary infections. Dietary supplements containing L-carnitine or acetyl-L-carnitine may be beneficial.
186	**Type**: Blood **Area**: Fatty Acid Metabolism **Marker**: Behetic	Low. Saturated fat. Very long chain fatty acids. Usually too high due to low physical exertion and high fat diet.
187	**Type**: Blood **Area**: Fatty Acid Metabolism **Marker**: Tricosanoic	High. Saturated fat. Points to vitamins B7, B12 or carnitine deficiency. Carnitine is required for fatty acid oxidation.
188	**Type**: Blood **Area**: Fatty Acid Metabolism **Marker**: Lignoceric	High. Saturated fat. Very long chain fatty acids. Usually too high due to low physical exertion and high fat diet.
189	**Type**: Blood **Area**: Fatty Acid Metabolism **Marker**: Pentadecanoic (Saturated)	High. Points to vitamins B7, B12 or carnitine deficiency. Carnitine is required for fatty acid oxidation.
190	**Type**: Blood **Area**: Fatty Acid Metabolism **Marker**: Saturated Fat %	Low. Fat from meat, dairy, coconuts, or palm oils. Can also point to vitamins B7, B12 or carnitine deficiency.

191	**Type**: Urine **Area**: Fatty Acid Metabolism **Marker**: Acetoacetic	Low. Ketones, such as 3-hydroxybutyric and acetoacetic acids, are the end-products of rapid or excessive fatty-acid breakdown. If elevated, points to prolonged fasting, protein malnutrition, high fat diet, vitamin B12 deficiency, severe GI Candida overgrowth, or pulmonary infections. Dietary supplements containing L-carnitine or acetyl-L-carnitine may be beneficial.
192	**Type**: Urine **Area**: Fatty Acid Metabolism **Marker**: 4-Hydroxybutyric	Low. A moderate urinary increase may be due to intake of dietary supplements containing 4-hydroxybutyric acid. Very high results may indicate a genetic disorder involving succinic semialdehyde dehydrogenase deficiency.
193	**Type**: Urine **Area**: Fatty Acid Metabolism **Marker**: Ethylmalonic	Low. Elevated levels can be due to carnitine deficiency, fasting, or increased intake of triglycerides from coconut oil, adipic acid containing Jell-O, or some infant formulas. Very elevated values may indicate a genetic disorder. Fatty acid oxidation defects are associated with hypoglycemia, and lethargy. Supplements L-carnitine, or acetyl-L-carnitine may help.
194	**Type**: Urine **Area**: Fatty Acid Metabolism **Marker**: Adipic Acid	High. Formed from "omega" oxidation of fats when beta oxidation is impaired due to deficiencies in vitamin B2 or carnitine, which impedes use by mitochondria. This may due to insufficient acetyl CoA (or its precursors cysteine, vitamin B5, magnesium), insulin excess, or ketosis. Can also point to excessive intake of gelatin or other "junk" food that has adipic acid additive.

195	**Type**: Urine **Area**: Fatty Acid Metabolism **Markers**: Suberic Acid and Sebacic acid	High. Formed from "omega" oxidation of fats when beta oxidation is impaired due to deficiencies in vitamin B2 or carnitine, which impedes use by mitochondria. Can indicate fat digestion issues, fasting, or increased intake of triglycerides from coconut oil, or some infant formulas. Very elevated values may indicate a genetic disorder. It can be associated with hypoglycemia and lethargy. L-carnitine, or acetyl-L-carnitine supplements may help.

CHAPTER THREE

Root Cause Hypothesis

My thoughts on the root cause of my pancreas damage. An insight into health issues caused by slow and long term deterioration due to chronic bodily insults, some of which you might not have considered before.

An example of the impact of the modern diet on the body, with its excessive sugar, pesticides, herbicides, chemicals, industrialized oils, toxic water, subsequent oxidative stress and microbiome dysbiosis. Its direct link to a myriad of modern health issues is staggering.

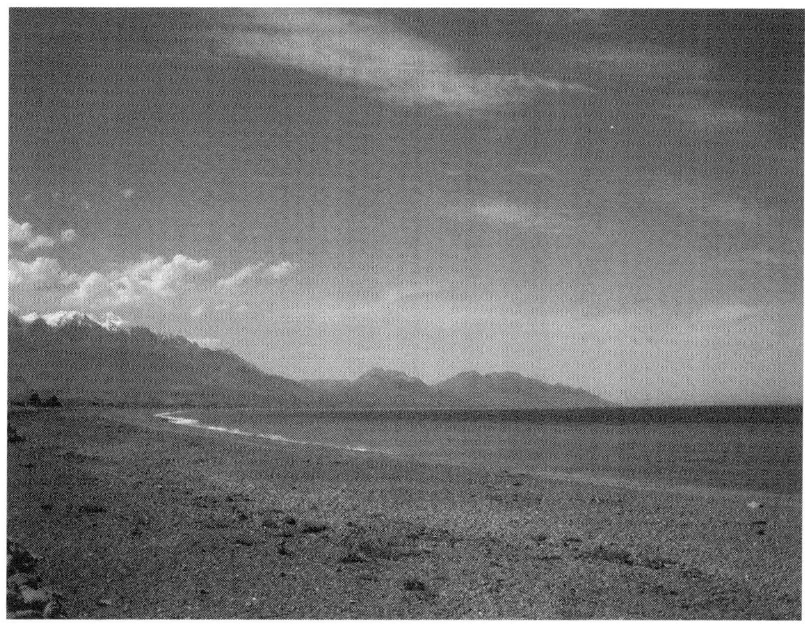

In school we were taught to ask "Why?" five times to get to the root cause of an issue. That practice is clearly lacking in today's Western medical system when it comes to chronic symptoms and illnesses.

I was never satisfied with the non-answers received from doctors, and was forced to continue asking the necessary discovery questions, determine which specialties might be relevant, find new doctors, request the necessary tests, and apply what I had learnt to become functional again.

As an IT consultant I was looking at my situation as buggy code that required fixing, and that included looking at inputs and outputs of the system, hardware and software issues. I needed to understand the root cause of the problem in order to fix it. Why do I feel so ill? How did this happen? Why did I get Chronic Fatigue Syndrome? Why did I get secondary mitochondrial dysfunction? Why did I get nutrient deficiencies? Why did I get exocrine pancreatic insufficiency? Why did my pancreas get damaged? I just had to keep digging further.

Many doctors stop at the nutrient deficiency question *if* they even test for it. For example, if a vitamin D test shows you are insufficient, the solution is to take some vitamin D supplements, or to get more sunshine. But why did you become deficient in the first place? Are you using up vitamin D too quickly in a specific metabolic pathway, perhaps due to too much insulin secretion or an overworked immune system? What stresses are you battling for which your body needs all that extra vitamin D? Are you not absorbing related cofactor nutrients properly? Why is that? EPI is just one possible reason for nutrient deficiencies, but rarely on the radar of a doctor. Damage to the exocrine pancreatic function causes issues with producing and releasing pancreatic enzymes into the duodenum at the right time and quantity. But how did you damage the pancreas in the first place?

If you are lucky, your doctor would have tested for vitamin D because you complained of fatigue and low energy, and that is as far as it went. This is exactly what happened with me and likely a similar story to many other sufferers out there. It was only years of suffering later that I understood that I was not breaking down fat properly due to my pancreas not releasing enough lipase enzymes. Since vitamin D is fat-soluble, I was not getting enough vitamin D through food. In addition, because of the excess sugar and oxidative stress burdens my body was continuously trying to overcome, I actually needed more vitamin D than usual. Oxidative stress was damaging my pancreas, and thus a vicious cycle had been occurring for all of those years. I just use vitamin D here as an illustration, but you can replace it with any vitamin, mineral, fatty acid or amino acid deficiency.

In hindsight, the root cause in my case is shockingly simple but with dreadful effects. This is all just based on my experiences and observations, not some rigorous large-scale scientific experiment. My own body was the experiment, both in terms of studying the negative effects of the toxins and oxidative stress overload of the modern Western diet and tap water, and the subsequent positive results when I removed those same insults and resolved the root cause.

Since a picture always helps, I will start with this summary diagram and then delve into the main points a little in separate subsections.

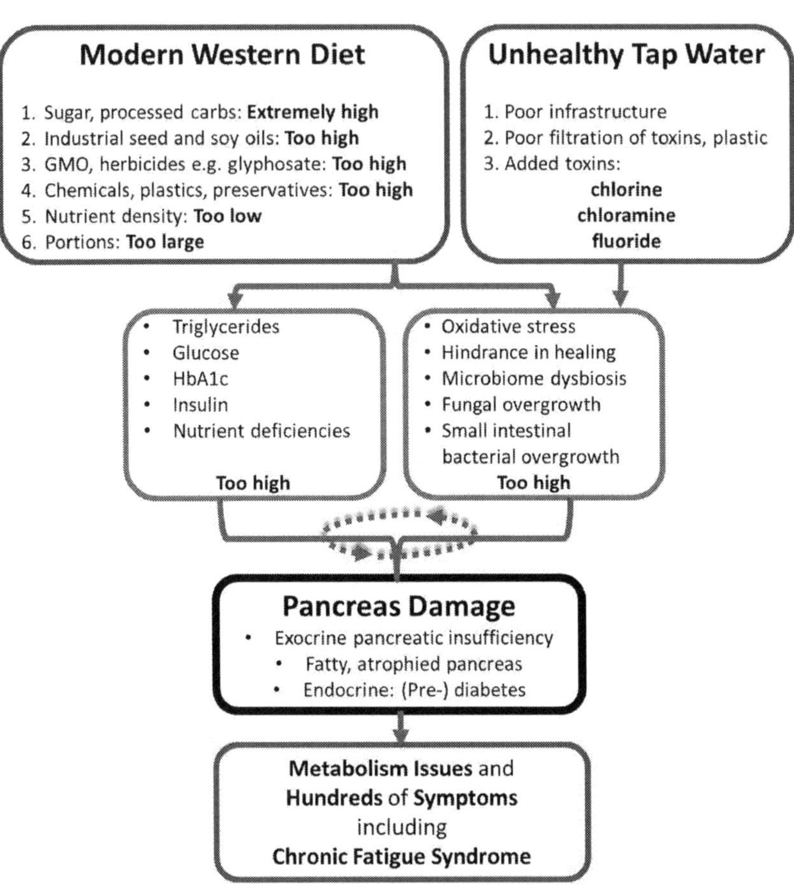

Diagram: Root cause hypothesis of my pancreatic damage

In my case, it was damage accumulated over two decades of exposure to the standard modern Western food supply. This included extreme levels of sugar, processed carbohydrates, industrialized seed oils, preventative added antibiotics, growth hormones, corn and soy fed animal products, with mostly GMO content and subsequent high levels of glyphosate, 2,4D and atrazine types of herbicides and pesticides. In addition, there was exposure to unhealthy tap water, with its added chlorine, ammonia, fluoride, and many other unfiltered toxins. All these bodily insults over time caused a number of vicious cycles, slowly damaging the pancreas and my health.

Possible Known Causes of EPI

There are a few standard causes of EPI such as:

- Pancreatitis (Chronic, autoimmune or acute)
- Pancreatic cancer
- Non-alcoholic fatty pancreas
- Atrophied pancreas
- Cystic fibrosis
- Duct obstructions
- Surgery of pancreatic or gastrointestinal functions
- Celiac or Crohn diseases
- Shwachman-Diamond or Johanson-Blizzard syndromes
- Zollinger-Ellison or Pearson-Marrow syndromes
- Alcohol
- Bacterial or viral

However, none of those more commonly known causes really explained *why* I ended up here.

Root Cause Hypothesis

The official medical cause of my non-alcoholic advanced fatty atrophy of the pancreas is still unknown. According to the literature, pancreatic atrophy could be due to, for example, chronic pancreatitis, alcoholism, hereditary, autoimmune, bacterial, viral or idiopathic reasons. Idiopathic, which is where my situation officially ended up, is just a fancy medical term for, "we have no clue".

Subsequent tests ruled out autoimmune, viruses and bacteria. Acute or chronic pancreatitis was ruled out since there was no visible scarring of the pancreas seen on the MRI. A hereditary cause was ruled out since no one else in the family has had any known exocrine pancreas issues.

With clean living, i.e., no drugs, no smoking, little alcohol and only in my younger years, only sporadic medicine for acute infections or headaches, very little fast food, no extreme stresses, lots of sports, healthy emotional and social life, in some ways I am as well a controlled experiment of the impact of the modern Western food supply on the body as you can find.

Even though I always thought I was eating a healthy balanced diet, low in sugar, few snacks and junk food, lots of vegetables, dairy, limited red meat, whole grains, I had no idea how atrocious the standard food industry and tap water quality really is. Large portion sizes, much traveling for work and subsequent eating in restaurants for many years really exacerbated the effect.

My root cause hypothesis as to the fundamental reason of my pancreatic damage is these insults and vicious cycles.

Insults

20 years of exposure to these insults destroyed most of my pancreas and seriously impacted my health:

1. Extreme levels of sugar and processed carbohydrates in food and drinks in its many different forms (e.g., HFCS), often from GMO/glyphosate/atrazine sources.

2. GMO/glyphosate/atrazine herbicides and chemicals treated industrial, highly processed seed (e.g., Canola), corn and soy oil.

3. GMO/glyphosate/atrazine herbicides treated vegetables and glyphosate herbicide sprayed modern wheat.

4. Meat, eggs and dairy from animals fed GMO/glyphosate/ atrazine treated soy and corn, and too much added antibiotics and growth hormones.

5. Unhealthy tap water quality with added toxic chemicals such as fluoride, chlorine and chloramine, as well as other toxins not sufficiently filtered out.

Vicious Cycles

These five insults subsequently caused vicious cycles in the following areas, further damaging the pancreas and my health:

1. **Oxidative stress**
2. **Microbiome dysbiosis**
3. **Pancreatic damage**
4. **Nutrient deficiencies**
5. **Hampered healing ability**

These five elements each reinforced the downward health spiral eventually leading to pre-EPI and EPI, the breakdown of the pancreas as well as the rest of my body over time. Microbiome dysbiosis increases nutrient deficiencies, oxidative stress, and hampers healing. Oxidative stress is essentially damaging (rusting) your body from the inside using up a lot of nutrients and hampering healing ability. Pancreatic damage is increased by nutrient deficiencies, which in turn causes more nutrient deficiencies, oxidative stress and microbiome dysbiosis. Your body tries very hard to stay in balance, but at some point it can no longer handle the negative impacts of the resulting vicious cycles.

Chronic exposure to low levels of a toxic substance causes oxidative stress and damages your health; it might just take a little longer!

Obviously, there is always a genetic factor involved, as in my case my pancreas was the weakest link in my body and the first to break. There are many people out there who have abused their body with alcohol, smoking, drugs and far worse food habits for longer than I have been alive, and they have no immediately evident issues with their pancreas. They might break something else first instead of the pancreas, or in the extreme outliers not be affected with illness. In my case, the first likely hit came from alcohol during my student days and partying in my early twenties. But, I drank far less than most of my peers, even during this time, and I never felt healthier than in my twenties. My pancreas could have also been weakened by a virus or bacteria during my world travels whilst growing up. But, the more important hit was the slow and constant assault of the modern Western food and tap water supply. "Death by a thousand cuts", to use the old saying.

Many others might be suffering from some form of pancreatic damage without really knowing this is the case, because it is so hard to establish, unless acute. The insults to your body can slowly deteriorate your health, and it can take many years before you start to feel and recognize the direct and indirect expanding effects. Since the pancreas is so sensitive of an organ, it is a good early warning indicator of the dangers of an unhealthy food supply. The immense and fast growing diabetes issue is confirmation of this, with the related exocrine issues currently flying under the radar, and vastly underreported at this time.

The factors I mentioned above are possibly the root cause for many modern illnesses, wherever modern food and agricultural supply and practices have been exported to. This includes nasties like obesity, metabolic disorder, hypertension, cardiovascular diseases, type 2 diabetes, heart diseases, atherosclerosis, autoimmune disease (e.g., Hashimoto's thyroid, rheumatoid arthritis, Lupus), food allergies and sensitivities, nutrient deficiencies, systemic inflammation, ME/CFS, gastrointestinal ailments (e.g., microbiome dysbiosis, SIBO, Candida, acid reflux, leaky gut, irritable bowel, Crohn's), hormone and fertility issues, pancreatic damage, neurotransmitter issues (e.g., depression, Alzheimer, anxiety, ADHD) and even many types of cancer. Many young children are now diagnosed with conditions like diabetes and obesity, previously rarely seen that young.

Standard Modern Western Diet

To be blunt, I was naïve and distinctly lacked knowledge on nutrition and the long term impact of food and water. I was yet another unwitting victim of the modern Western food supply. The standard American diet (SAD), or rather the standard Western or standard modern diet, is spreading rapidly across the globe and bringing with it many modern ailments.

A few of the standard themes are familiar:

1. Large portions of food that have increased considerably over the years, thus causing a high surplus in daily calories.

2. Massively sized, and also growing, sugary drinks.

3. High levels of processed foods.

4. Lots of dairy and red meat.

5. Lots of packaged food and drinks.

6. Too little fresh produce, fresh fish and real whole grains.

7. Plenty of 24/7 available cheap fast food.

8. Instant and microwave meals.

9. Lots of restaurant and store bought meals.

10. Not enough time allocated or available to buy fresh food and prepare at home.

11. Convenience and price versus quality and time.

12. High AGE level. Foods containing high levels of advanced glycation end products (AGE).

However, this list is missing a few key elements that are perhaps a little less obvious, but not less damaging to our health.

Additional Modern Western Diet Health Impacts:

13. Extreme levels of GMO, glyphosate and atrazine type herbicides sprayed sugar and chemical sugar substitutes in all its varied forms, often used as a cheap preservative.

14. GMO, glyphosate and atrazine sprayed food products. This used to be a North American centric issue, but has spread to the rest of the globe. Even in Europe, GMO is hidden in the form of imported animal feed, processed and packaged foods, and fast food chain ingredients.

15. GMO, glyphosate and atrazine sprayed animal feed.

16. Industrialized seed oils marketed as "vegetable oil" are used in almost everything, and are mostly GMO, herbicide sprayed, highly processed and unhealthy. For example, GMO soybean oil usage is widespread, and surprisingly an important contributor to diabetes.

17. Widespread preventative use of antibiotics in animals we eat.

18. Growth hormones used in some of the animals we eat.

19. The bad reputation of red meat and dairy these days is focusing on the wrong elements as to why they can be unhealthy. Sure, the portions are often ridiculous, but it is the industrialized, inhumane, feedlot, factory-style farming that is non-organic, full of antibiotics and GMO, glyphosate and atrazine sprayed animal feed that is the real cause of concern.

20. Tap water with nasty toxins that are not filtered out sufficiently and additional toxins that are added in, such as chlorine, chloramines and fluoride. This helps kill good gut bacteria, in addition to causing your body to work overtime in trying to cope with filtering out the toxins.

21. Wheat and wheat products are in almost everything packaged, as it is a cheap filler. It is often stripped of all the healthy micronutrients since the wheat germ has a very short shelf life. This leaves just the starch, which is just glucose to your body. In North America wheat is allowed to be chemically bleached. Wheat gets a bad reputation these days, and the increase in availability of gluten-free products shows how people have grown more sensitive and intolerant to wheat products. But again, the focus is on the wrong area. Wheat is often sprayed with glyphosate type herbicides in order to speed up the harvesting process, which lowers important minerals and reduces important essential amino acids from the wheat. It cannot be washed off, so the antibiotic is ingested with the wheat. Modern day wheat is a hybridized version that is very different from even 50 years ago. People's beneficial bacteria are under constant attack from various sources when they are actually essential in being able to break down gluten! So you eat glyphosate (with its antibiotic effect) rich wheat products, killing the good bacteria you actually need to break down those same wheat products.

22. Chemical additives overload. Used for anything from anticaking, emulsifiers (food glue), preservatives, coloring, flavor enhancers, to texture and appearance. This causes health issues such as oxidative stress and autoimmune reactions.

23. Plastics exposure from almost all food products including to-go drink cups, packaging, soup and soda cans (plastic lining), cartons, water bottles, straws, etc. In many coffee chains it is difficult to get coffee in glass or ceramic instead of the plastic (yes most "paper" cups contain a lining of plastic or other chemicals!) or polystyrene ones. You ingest plastic particles as well as leached chemicals like phthalates, BPA, BPF, BPS, PFC, or PVC. And, I am only talking about the direct health impact of the plastic, not the secondary environmental impact through the disposal of all that plastic in the oceans and water supplies. It is now found in most tap water and ocean sourced fish.

24. Unreasonable fear of bacteria, which causes behavior that kills our essential good bacteria in the body, with massive subsequent

health impacts. With all the antimicrobial soaps, sprays and wipes, antibiotics in meat, antibiotics (through glyphosate) sprayed on crops, overprescribing of antibiotics, there is this almost phobic misunderstanding of bacteria, and lack of knowledge on how essential the beneficial ones are for our health.

25. "Just eat healthy food". Yes, but what does that mean exactly? Many people lack this food knowledge, or think that they are eating healthily, like I was. Incorrect and unhealthy messages are spread through overwhelming and dishonest marketing, packaging, sponsored pseudo-health institutions, and lack of food education. Doctors get very limited nutritional education. Perhaps this is due to big industry's financial involvement in politics, medical education and research? The food pyramid, which is how many kids are fed in schools, was altered by the food industry to become not only not healthy, but actually detrimental to health.

All of the above help destroy the essential good microbiota in the body and cause microbiome dysbiosis. The microbiome protects us from disease and nasty bacteria, supports the immune system, aids the breakdown of food into necessary nutrients, produces vitamins, helps prevent infections and has been linked to lower symptoms of inflammatory bowel disease and even cardiovascular illnesses. Happily, this field of research into the impacts of the microbiome on our health has been gaining in strength and popularity.

In addition, the exposure to toxic metals, preservatives, chemicals, plastics, herbicides and pesticides cause our antioxidant system to be overwhelmed, causing oxidative stress and subsequent breakdowns in the body.

Nutritional Deserts and Cheap Food

A while ago I read the term "nutritional desert" and thought it was spot on. There is indeed a problem of a lack of nutrients in the standard modern Western diet. This has multiple causes which were mentioned above, from the many artificial ingredients, industrial farming, soil micronutrient depletion, herbicides and pesticides usage, lack of time and effort around food, lack of food education, to the lack of whole, fresh food. But there are areas in the United States, for example, that are called "nutritional deserts" since people have no *affordable* options to get fresh organic produce and healthy restaurant food. Instead they are confronted with strip mall after another of nutritionally deficient, sugar excessive, harmful, processed, chain and fast food.

When your body sends you the message of hunger, or a craving, it is telling you it needs, not just macronutrients for energy, but also micronutrients. By eating more of the same nutrient-poor food this craving does not go away. People will continue to snack as well as increase portion sizes to try to fill this craving, and end up taking in too many "empty calories". Packaged goods and fast food manufacturers play into this by designing and marketing their products to get you to eat more. It still does not alleviate the nutrient craving signal your body is sending you.

This can then lead to nutrient deficiencies, with constant fatigue and low energy as some resulting symptoms. It is no coincidence that coffee shops and energy drink sales are through the roof. People need stimulants to get extra energy, since many are not getting enough micronutrients from food. Those drinks are an easy hit to get you through the day, but are often sugar excessive and devoid of any nutrients.

Most restaurants use excessive amounts of sugar, corn and soy-fed meat, seed and soybean oils. These are cheap, mostly non-organic, GMO and thus generously sprayed with glyphosate and atrazine types of herbicides. It is all in the name of profits.

People look for the cheapest food to eat and produce, with long shelf lives (i.e., through chemicals and sugars), but there really are no shortcuts. You eat because you need nutrients to keep your metabolic pathways functioning, and avoid breakdowns and disease. Strangely, the fewer the ingredients, the more expensive the product. Meat is bulked up and grown as quickly as possible, through high sugar content feed that was grown quickly using lots of pesticides and herbicides, not to mention all the added antibiotics. Vegetables, fruits and grains agriculture is similarly sped up through practices that require immense amounts of nutrient leaching pesticides and herbicides. There is often not enough time for it to ripen naturally and produce adequate nutrients (e.g., essential amino acids) that we, and the animals we eat, need.

You pay now (more for slow, organic food) or you will pay later (more medical bills and lost income). The latter is sadly becoming sooner and sooner these days. For those over thirty or forty, how many people do you know in your direct surroundings that have some sort of ailment for which they are taking medicine, or other types of supplementation? We have to rely more and more on antibiotics or antivirals to fight off even small infections, when the primary cause was not having a balanced microbiome and immune system, and the necessary nutrients to fight it naturally. Many people are taking antidepressants and painkillers these days, when a major core cause is the lack of nutrients necessary to produce the necessary neurotransmitters. The chlorinated water and glyphosate rich food is also contributing to microbiome dysbiosis. Many children these days are microbiome imbalanced and nutritionally deficient, likely causing symptoms like ADHD, aggression and depression. Children are being pumped full of hardcore medicines and mood altering drugs, when rarely is the quality of food and drink, excessive sugar and the nutrient deficiencies looked at as a root cause. Cheap food!

Modern "Healthy" Lunch Example

But, what is healthy nutritious food? I used to think I was eating a healthy lunch by ordering wheat bread, pasta with chicken and a salad at a restaurant until I understood what that mostly meant. Here is an example of my lack of knowledge at the time:

- **Chicken**. Chlorine washed and GMO/glyphosate/atrazine corn and soy fed. Who knew you had to ask for air-chilled, organic, and pasture-raised to get decent chicken meat?

- **Vegetables**. GMO/glyphosate/atrazine sprayed vegetables drenched in sugary industrial soy, corn or rapeseed oil dressing.

- **Pasta**. GMO/glyphosate sprayed bleached wheat, stripped of its nutrients for shelf life, with sauce from non-organic ingredients, high in processed carbs and sugar for preservative.

- **Vegetable oil**. This is a misnomer as it does not contain any vegetables, but is usually GMO/glyphosate/atrazine seed (Canola), corn or soy oil.

- **Salt**. Standard table salt is often bleached, without any of the good minerals in it, with added sugar (dextrose) and silicate, or other anti-caking agents.

- **Water, coffee or tea**. Exposure to unhealthy water quality with inadequate filtering of toxins and added ones like chlorine, fluoride and chloramines.

- **To-go**. Due to work pressure I often took food and coffee take-out, not knowing about the amount of added exposure to toxins from food wrappers, boxes, styrene, cups, plastics, etc.

It is not just a North American problem, as Europe has raced towards the same model with food and agriculture practices. There are a few lonely holdouts slowly succumbing to pressure, where big business dictates the direction of a country's laws and health. It is often stealthily done. Ingredients are substituted for cheaper GMO or artificial kinds. Seemingly strict European GMO laws are circumvented by importing GMO soy and corn as animal feed, or in a processed form. Tastes are slowly changed so that more sugar can be used as a cheap preservative. Shelf lives of products have increased drastically by adding more sugar and chemicals, to the detriment of health, in order to boost profits. Many people actually have pointed out that certain snacks, cookies or chips of the same brand used to taste much better a few decades ago. Just to give another indication of the trend, in Holland, where modern ailments have also been growing leaps and bounds in the last decade, there is now a ten percent diabetes rate. This is already a stunning rise compared to when I grew up there. But, let's look at the effects of sugar a little more.

Excess Sugar and Processed Carbs

Excess sugar and processed carbs can cause serious damage to the pancreas, both on the endocrine and exocrine sides. The extreme level of sugar of all types and in all kinds of products, even those for young kids and infants, is truly scary. There are many ways that sugar is marketed differently on the packaging to make it seem healthier. There is even rampant and nefarious marketing directed at children, making excessive levels of sugar seem normal and desirable! It is used in huge amounts as a cheap preservative. Ever wondered why most supermarket bread, condiments, packaged foods, or a hamburger from many of the fast food chains stays the same when left out for weeks or months?

Restaurants are using an insane amount of sugar and processed carbs in everything. I am not even talking about the usual fast food chain suspects, but even many restaurants and cafés which pretend to be healthy are really just diabetes and inflammation factories. Just check out the nutrient listing on their website and you will be shocked to see how, for example, one vegetable dish you thought was healthy contains more sugar than you should eat in a week. You have to carefully read nutrition labels and familiarize yourself with all the various ways manufacturers list sugar using innocent looking names.

It is truly disgusting how the profits of corporations are more important than the health of a population, including small children. Just look up the nefarious sugar research reports from the 1950s for which we are as a society still paying the price. You can read how difficult it is for even governments to change a simple thing, like packaging to warn consumers of high levels of sugar, or to stop companies from advertising to small children through the use of cuddly animals and cartoons. Marketing along with its deceiving packaging and labeling has been so successful that kids and adults think the following example is a healthy breakfast.

Modern Breakfast Example

- **Cereal**. Copious amounts of GMO sugar, chemicals, glyphosate rich and nutrient-poor bleached wheat, oats or atrazine sprayed GMO corn. The wheat is often without any of the micronutrient rich wheat germ, as that spoils quickly and thus impedes shelf life and profit.

- **More sugar** sprinkled on top of the cereal, perhaps in the perceived healthier form of honey, brown sugar, maple or agave syrup.

- **Non-fat cow milk.** Lots of sugar in the form of tough to break down lactose, without the fat to help keep the insulin spike in check. Often sourced from GMO/glyphosate/atrazine corn and soy fed cows plied with growth hormones and antibiotics. It is made to seem healthier by fortifying it with vitamin A and D. There are better ways to get your vitamins and calcium. Organic grass-fed cow milk is better since it has higher omega-3 and linoleic acid levels and fewer nasties. Milk substitutes are often highly processed, with added ingredients, and GMO/glyphosate sprayed products like soymilk which are touted as healthy.

- **Fruit juices.** Huge amounts of sugar, chemicals, and often sourced abroad. Those that are advertised as "no added sugar" will still provide excess sugar. Even a glass of freshly squeezed orange juice requires more oranges than you should have in a whole week. It is a terribly inefficient and unhealthy way to get your vitamin C.

- **White bread or bagel** should be considered cake, as it contains more sugar per slice than a whole loaf should have. Glyphosate rich, nutrient-poor, bleached wheat, often without the wheat germ, and with added chemicals. This is topped with high sugar content peanut butter and high fructose corn syrup jelly with some coloring. It still amazes me to see the huge aisles of "plastic", chemically smelling bread in the supermarkets, that stay the same for months as even mold and bacteria do not fancy it. Proper bread should not last longer than one to two days before going bad, should contain wheat germ and bran, and the only sugar used should be the tiny bit needed to bring the yeast to life, if need be.

• **Deli meats**. Often from GMO/glyphosate/atrazine herbicide sprayed and antibiotics fed animals with added chemicals, nitrite, and a surprisingly large amount of sugar as a cheap preservative.

Modern Snacking Examples

Add to this the abundance of snacks and drinks often enjoyed during the day, which provide more hits of chemicals, refined carbs and GMO sugar. People have become so accustomed to excess sugar levels that they forget how little is healthy and how much they are actually taking in each day. A few examples:

• Bucket sized soda (a *small* size is often almost 0.5 liter or 16 fluid ounces!), energy drinks, sports drinks, tea drinks, fast food, microwave meals, and most packaged snacks.

• One "small" (0.5l) soda contains more than double, the World Health Organization (WHO) recommended daily adult intake of sugar. Orange juice has almost the same amount of sugar.

• A tablespoon of ketchup contains a teaspoon of sugar.

• Troughs of sugary and milky coffee drinks

• Sugar laden and processed carb heavy products that are marketed or perceived as healthy, such as fruit shakes, smoothies, granola, dried fruit, cereals, protein and nut bars, vegetable drinks, trail mix, flavored or frozen yoghurt, etc.

Just because something is labelled organic, gluten-free, natural, low-fat, diet, reduced sugar does not mean it actually contains healthy amounts of sugar. Read the labels and it might surprise you. And remember that the body procceses carbs into glucose.

It is little wonder so many kids are obese and diabetic, and arthritis or an autoimmune disease starting in your twenties is not uncommon. Alzheimer rates are spiking, and it is sometimes referred to as "diabetes 3" by its link to long term insulin resistance, where at some point the brain can no longer use glucose for energy well. To make things even worse was the low-fat, high-carb diet craziness of the last decades, which luckily seems to have finally turned a corner.

More than a third of the US population is either pre- or full-blown diabetic. Of those with diabetes around twenty-five to fifty percent will likely also have exocrine pancreatic damage, according to some studies. But many people are undiagnosed, and just suffering the consequences of excess sugar.

Whether it is called agave syrup, honey, dextrose, fructose, corn syrup, fruit juice, lactose, milk powder, cane sugar or juice, ethyl maltol, caramel, glucose, malt, maltodextrin, sorbitol, treacle, molasses, or natural sweetener, it will impact your pancreas and the oxidative stress effects on the body.

Excess Blood Sugar (Glucose) Effect on the Body

Often too many grams of carbs are consumed per meal. And, on average twenty percent of daily calories are now consumed through sugar, when not long ago in human history that percentage was negligible. Many books have been written on the effects that high carbs and sugar have on the body, so I will just highlight a few points linking the effect on pancreatic damage:

- **Oxidative Stress**. Excess sugar leads to the forming of excess reactive oxygen species (ROS), which then gets into a vicious cycle of triggering even more ROS. When the generation of ROS in the body exceeds the ability to neutralize the damage through the body's amazing antioxidant systems, cell damage (i.e., oxidative stress) occurs.

• **Glycation** is the bonding of a sugar molecule to a fat or protein molecule without the need of an enzyme to perform this process, which can happen either in the body or outside the body. Excess sugar causes advanced glycation end products (AGE), which can lead to reactive oxygen species (ROS) and oxidative stress.

• **Mitochondrial reactive oxygen species** (ROS) creation imbalance also occurs with excess glucose metabolism (Glycolysis) or impaired oxidative phosphorylation (OxPhos). This can lead to mitochondrial dysfunction and ultimately cell death.

• **Insulin spikes** and **resistance**, **diabetes** and **pre-diabetes**. Your body understands that glucose needs to be utilized and cannot be in the blood at high levels for long before doing damage. Insulin will inhibit the body from using fat as energy, so that glucose in the blood will be used and thus lowered. However, too much glucose, followed by too much insulin, and over time cells become resistant to the effects of insulin. The pancreas will try to produce even more insulin to try to lower the blood glucose. The liver is impacted due to increasing glycogen stores.

• **Vitamin D** is required for insulin secretion. Excess sugar is likely an important, but not often discussed, reason for the widespread vitamin D insufficiencies seen these days.

• **Excess sugar and carbs are turned into triglycerides** in the liver, which is then stored as fat, including in the liver and pancreas; impacting the functioning of those organs. I had many years of unhealthy triglyceride levels. It was my body's message that I was consuming too much sugar and processed carbohydrates, resulting in visceral fat deposits particularly in the pancreas. Non-alcoholic fatty liver disease, another fast rising health issue, and non-alcoholic fatty pancreas share this root cause.

Some may think that extremely high levels of triglycerides are needed, but I am a perfect example of how just elevated triglyceride levels cause slow but serious damage over time!

Also, just because the average triglyceride levels have increased drastically in the last twenty to thirty years does not mean humans have genetically changed to make this normal or healthy. Fatty atrophy was perhaps a defense mechanism of my body to try to avoid even worse, and try to heal from the excess glucose intake and its oxidative stress. High triglycerides will also cause higher levels of LDL (low-density lipoprotein). A few more sugar points:

• **Fructose** is often added to products as a sweetener, metabolizes into fat and is handled by the liver in similar fashion to alcohol. High fructose corn syrup (HFCS) is widely used.

• **Excess sugar also feeds yeast** (e.g., Candida) and causes dysbiosis in the microbiome, where the balance between good and bad bacteria and yeast is out of sync.

• **Chronic Fatigue Syndrome** is another possible effect of long term excess sugar, as it is tied to oxidative stress and mitochondrial dysfunction.

• **GMO and herbicides.** Most sugar in North America is made from GMO corn, GMO sugar beets or GMO sugar cane, all of which are generously sprayed with herbicides like glyphosate and atrazine. A double whammy to the body!

Industrialized Seed Oils

Vegetable oils used in most packaged goods and almost every single restaurant, even the fancy ones, are a misnomer. They are *not* made of vegetables at all, but instead are mostly GMO, glyphosate herbicide sprayed, chemically processed, micronutrient and phytonutrient reduced, seed, cotton or soybean oils. Another favorite is corn oil, which is mostly GMO and in North America sprayed with atrazine, an endocrine disruptor.

It is important to consume omega-3 (abundant in, e.g., fish oils, grass-fed protein), omega-9 (abundant in, e.g., olive oil) and omega-6 (abundant in, e.g., grains, seeds, nuts) for your health, but it needs to be balanced. The consumption ratio of omega-6 to omega-3 is often highly skewed in the modern Western diet, with omega-6 often ten to twenty times higher than omega-3. This ratio should not be higher than 4-to-1 and closer to 1-to-1 to be healthy. Not omega-6 by itself, as it is essential, but the excess intake and the source of the omega-6 is what causes inflammation and subsequent health issues over time.

Soybean oil, one of the biggest omega-6 sources these days and used everywhere, is an important contributor to diabetes. Canola, which is mostly from GMO, glyphosate sprayed, chemically processed rapeseed, is not that good for you, no matter what the marketing machine tells you. They are heated, bleached, deodorized, and treated with chemicals like hexane in the production process. Industrial seed oils are very high in omega-6 in relation to omega-3. They contain low levels of trans-fats which are far higher than in olive oil, for example.

Trans-fats were in the news quite a bit and there has been a push against them, but when you read "partially hydrogenated" on packaging that means that there is a good chance it contains trans-fats. Companies are allowed to market oil as "zero trans-fat" if a serving has less than 0.5 grams of trans-fats in it.

Really, olive oil (the non-fake, cold pressed, extra virgin kind) is the best one to use, with avocado and coconut also good for a slight bit of variation. Butter or ghee from organic grass-fed cows is also a good option for variety. Of course consume in moderation, and be aware of the temperature when cooking, as oils have different smoking points. This is the point at which oil starts to break down and release harmful chemicals, such as unhealthy fumes and advanced glycation end-products (AGE). This will then contribute to oxidative stress and inflammation.

GMO, Herbicides, Nutrient Deficient Food

Most crops in North America are now GMO, however, GMO by itself is likely a red herring. More important to consider is that

GMO goes together with excessive exposure to herbicides like 2,4D (2,4-Dichlorophenoxyacetic Acid), atrazine and glyphosate based ones. GMO essentially means that it can be sprayed with even more herbicides and pesticides without killing the plant.

The negative impact atrazine and glyphosate type herbicides have had, and still have, on health is not to be underestimated. When I mention "glyphosate" I mean the concoction of chemicals that make up a glyphosate based herbicide. For example, in a study I read it mentioned that the body's mitochondrial oxidative phosphorylation (i.e., energy generation) process was impacted negatively, not just by glyphosate itself, but the cell's membrane permeability was impacted by other chemicals in the herbicide.

You can look at the timing and increased usage of GMO, atrazine and glyphosate type herbicides through the various countries in the last few decades, and see the correlation of spikes in rates of diabetes, obesity, intestinal issues and autoimmune diseases. Of course we are taught that correlation does not imply causation, but the following points are intriguing:

1. Chelates minerals. Glyphosate was first patented as a chelating or descaling agent to remove minerals in order to keep water pipes and boilers clear of mineral build up. It can do the same in our food supply by binding to essential minerals, thus lowering crucial mineral levels of e.g., calcium, iron, magnesium, zinc, molybdenum, manganese, cobalt, selenium and copper in our food and animal feed. By leaching key mineral nutrients from the plant, I read that it can even interfere with the plant's photosynthesis and chlorophyll levels.

2. Antimicrobial. Glyphosate was then patented as an antimicrobial. It is an antibiotic which kills bacteria. It can do the same to gut bacteria, causing microbiome dysbiosis in both humans, and the animals we eat. Our good bacteria are needed in such functions as vitamin production (e.g., some B vitamins), metabolic, hormonal, immunity, neurotransmitter activity, and even in digestion, by helping to break down gluten and lactose.

3. Herbicide. Glyphosate was then patented as an herbicide, and is now the most widely used herbicide in the world. Not only is it used as a non-specific herbicide, it is also used in other cost-cutting processes such desiccating, which is the quick ripening or drying of crops. It penetrates the soil and plant and cannot be washed off before eating.

4. Disrupts amino acid production. As an herbicide, glyphosate disrupts the enzymes of the Shikimate metabolic pathway in plants, fungus and bacteria. This is used in the biosynthesis of folates, and the aromatic amino acids phenylalanine, tyrosine and tryptophan. Animals, including humans, do not have this metabolic pathway. Phenylalanine and tryptophan are essential amino acids that cannot be produced by our bodies or by the animals we eat. They are therefore considered essential amino acids and must be taken in through food.

5. Animal feed. The animals we eat are also impacted, since they are fed GMO, and thus glyphosate and atrazine sprayed feed. Ideally cows should only eat grass and chickens should only eat insects, without exposure to herbicides and pesticides. Instead they are fed herbicide rich, micronutrient-poor, amino acid (phenylalanine, tyrosine and tryptophan) poor feed, which can also impact their beneficial gut bacteria. This means they require more artificial supplementation. They also have a harder time fighting infections due to microbiome dysbiosis, and require more antibiotics. This impacts us not only through the meat we eat, but also eggs, milk, cheese and other dairy products.

6. Seeds and herbicide. GMO seeds and herbicides are often patented and sold by the same company. GMO really just means that those plants are able to handle far larger quantities of herbicides without dying, so that more can be used on increasingly herbicide resistant weeds.

7. Probable carcinogen. The World Health Organization called glyphosate a probable human carcinogen. California added it to the list of chemicals known to cause cancer under Proposition 65.

8. Endocrine disruptor. Atrazine is an herbicide that is an endocrine disruptor which affects, for example, hormones in humans and animals. It also easily contaminates the water supply and has been illegal in the European Union since 2003. However, it is one of the most used herbicides in North America and is used on most non-organic corn. This corn is fed to all non-organic cows, from which many people get their meat, dairy and milk. Much of the GMO sugar is corn based, with high fructose corn syrup used in many products.

There is a lot of noise surrounding this topic, and a lot of money is spent on marketing, lawyers, biased research and anti-studies. However, there are some great articles available and I am grateful to all the authors, researchers, scientists, farmers that are speaking out about this issue and sharing their data. I have listed a few links in the Appendix if you would like to delve deeper into the murky waters that is glyphosate and other herbicides. It is getting more news coverage of late due to litigation.

Oxidative Stress

In a simplistic analogy I picture oxidative stress as rust building up and damaging the cells and organs in the body. Collect enough rust in certain places and body parts start to break down. Oxidative stress can cause health issues such as neurodegenerative diseases, cardiovascular diseases, DNA mutations, cancers, Chronic Fatigue Syndrome, mitochondrial dysfunctions, and atrophy of the acinar cells of the pancreas.

Our body naturally produces reactive oxygen species (ROS) either through mitochondrial ATP energy production, detoxification of environmental toxins, or immune system functions. A subset of ROS are the highly reactive molecules known as free radicals, which are those with unpaired electrons. Normally, your body strives for a tightly controlled homeostasis, where antioxidants balance the free radicals. This is a normal part of a well-functioning body. However, when the amount of free radicals becomes excessive, the antioxidant mechanisms of the cell can become overwhelmed, leading to impaired cell function. In addition, if antioxidants in the food are too low, or nutrients and cofactors are lacking in order to produce the necessary antioxidants in the body, it can also lead to impaired cell function.

This imbalance is called oxidative stress, where this excess of free radicals damages cells in the body. Free radicals are looking for potential targets to bind ("steal" an electron) with. Without enough antioxidants, they can bind with membrane lipids, causing damage to cell walls, or proteins, leading to enzyme inactivation or receptor malfunction, or DNA, leading to mutations and potential cancers.

The usual suspects such as smoking, alcohol, drugs and toxin exposure, but also excess sugar and nutrient deficiencies cause excess free radicals in the body. Your body tries very hard to handle continuous oxidative stress from burning excess sugar and handling herbicides, pesticides, chlorine, fluoride, heavy metals and other toxins. With EPI it gets hit doubly hard by nutrient deficiencies, making it difficult to generate enough antioxidants to battle the effects. A simple, visual effect of free radical damage is age spots (a.k.a. liver spots) on the skin. It is usually linked to age, but also affects those much younger with high accumulative damage, as they are showing the effects of lipid oxidation.

Glutathione, glutathione peroxidase, superoxide dismutase (SOD), catalase and thioredoxin are all essential antioxidants produced in the body. Some of the well-known ones in food and supplements include glutathione, CoQ10, vitamins A, C and E. Glutathione enzymes require sufficient cofactors to function including vitamins C, E, B1, B2, B6, B9, selenium, magnesium, zinc, alpha lipoic acid (ALA). In addition, amino acids cysteine, glutamate and glycine are essential in the production of glutathione. CoQ10 can also be synthesized in the body if cofactors are sufficient. Anyone with any nutrient absorption and deficiency issues like EPI, Pre-EPI, SIBO, microbiome imbalance, or yeast overgrowth will have an issue with handling oxidative stress damage. This means your body is slowly "rusting" from the inside and at some point your weakest link breaks.

Vitamin D might also affect the production of glutathione according to some studies, however, this link is not confirmed at this time. It might be an indirect link due to the excessive sugar consumption requiring extra vitamin D for all the additional insulin secretion. BH4 is an essential cofactor in the synthesis of neurotransmitters and is highly sensitive to oxidation. It is rapidly destroyed by oxidative stress, which can lead to deficiencies in tyrosine, serotonin, dopamine, norepinephrine, and nitric oxide.

For those with pancreas damage, such as EPI and pre-EPI sufferers it becomes a vicious cycle. Oxidative stress causes destruction of the pancreas cells, which leads to not being able to absorb your food properly, leading to nutrient deficiencies, an inability to absorb and produce enough antioxidants, thus more oxidative stress, and eventually more pancreatic damage.

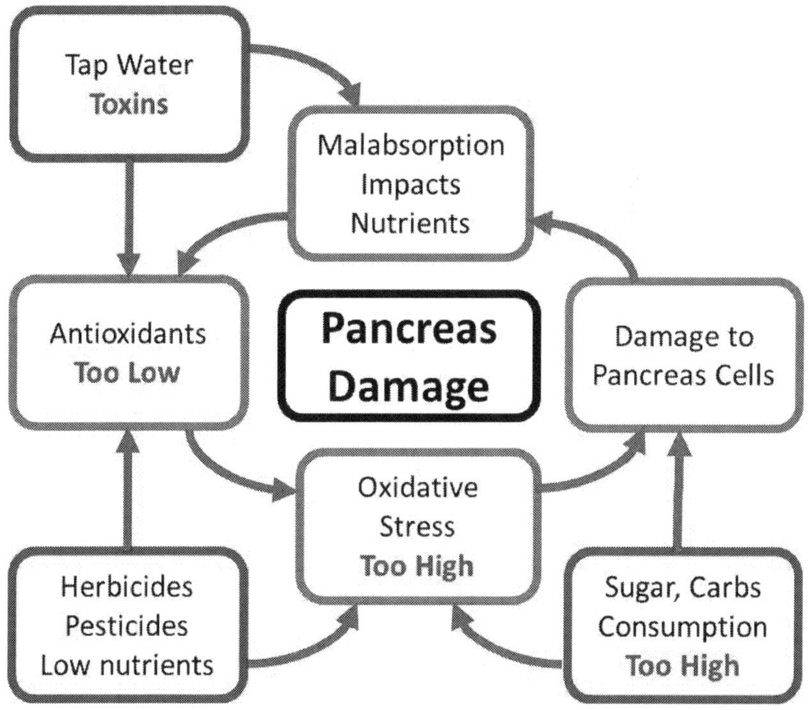

Diagram: Oxidative stress and pancreas damage vicious cycle

Tap Water Quality

This is an important and often overlooked element in the overall picture of health, healing, nutrient deficiencies, malabsorption and Chronic Fatigue Syndrome. Because you consume quite a bit of water daily and depend on it, this is a key area to scrutinize. It also provides many essential minerals, electrolytes, and trace elements. You need to pay attention to every contact with tap water, whether it is through hot or cold drinks, restaurant water, ice cubes, cooking, shower or bath contact.

The tap water supply in North America is surprisingly unhealthy in many cities, and likely a large contributor to many health issues. This can also include unlikely links such as obesity, food sensitivities, irritable bowel syndrome, acid reflux and autoimmune diseases. Some examples made it into international news, like Flint (Michigan), Erin Brockovich, or the flammable tap water stories due to the oil and gas fracking.

The general EPA approved water quality would not be considered acceptable in some parts of the world, and not just due to the levels of toxins that have not been filtered out properly, but the unhealthy additives. Chlorine, chloramine and fluoride are added to the water supply. The EPA even sets a minimum level of free chlorine that tap water needs to have when leaving the water treatment plant. Chlorine is added because it kills bacteria, but it also releases carcinogenic disinfection compounds like trihalomethanes and haloacetic acids. It is cheaper to just add more chlorine and chloramine, instead of using similar water treatment processes that are successfully used in other countries. Fixing the water supply distribution pipelines, so that there is less chance of pathogenic bacteria entering in transit from the treatment plant to your house, is perhaps seen as too costly. But the cost of this "cheap" method should really also include the overall health impact costs as well as lost income costs to society.

These additives cause microbiome dysbiosis by also killing your beneficial bacteria, with all the subsequent health issues. In addition, your body's antioxidant system, liver and kidneys have to work hard to clear out the toxins from the water, causing an additional drain on important nutrients. To give another example of a differing quality threshold, allowable levels of glyphosate in drinking water is 0.1 ppb (or micro gram/L) in Holland, but in the United States, the EPA allows for 700 ppb.

Fluoride is a toxin which we are constantly exposed to when drinking unfiltered tap water. Fluoride is used to kill rodents and termites. It can cause bone disease, brain and thyroid cell issues, mitochondrial dysfunction, oxidative stress, and neurotransmitter issues to list a few. The often mentioned benefit of fluoride additive to prevent tooth decay is nonsense. People in North Europe do not have more tooth decay than in North America. There is a reason it was outlawed decades ago as a tap water additive in most of Europe. In North America it is added mostly as hazardous waste from the fertilizer industry, in the form of hydrofluorosilicic acid (HFSA). The argument that the amount in tap water is too low to be damaging is not believable, and just as damaging an argument as the herbicides in food discussion.

Examples of a mostly unmonitored set of man-made toxins are the per- or poly-fluorinated chemicals (PFC) such as perfluorooctane sulfonate (PFOS) and perfluorooctanoic acid (PFOA). These are found in manufacturing plants, airports, consumer products such as non-stick pans, waterproof products, grease repellant products, food packaging and wrappers, and sadly in the tap water of many cities. There is also the relatively new issue with tap water, which is the amount of different types of micro-plastics that are not filtered out. The levels in US tap water were measured as one of the most contaminated in the world.

Chronic exposure to low levels of a toxic substance will cause oxidative stress and damage your health; it might just take a little longer!

Those people with EPI, CFS, or any health issues for that matter already have a tough enough time functioning and healing. Unhealthy tap water is an additional blow to the body that you do not need.

Sadly, there are not many *affordable* options available. Many people in my surroundings avoid tap water due to the taste, which in and of itself is a big hint your body is giving you. Instead, they rely on plastic water bottles or a home delivery service. Plastic bottles are another bad idea, with recent research showing that all water bottles contain small plastic particles that you consume. The much touted BPA-free slogan pertains to just one of the chemicals leaching in your water through plastic exposure. Others use carbon filters in water pitchers, fridges or even expensive installed ones under the kitchen sink. These filters take out much of the chlorine and perhaps some of the chloramine, but not many other nasties like fluoride and arsenic.

The very expensive reverse osmosis (RO) systems remove the most, but also remove much of the essential minerals that we need, in addition to wasting a lot of water in the process. There are many water shops in my area where people fill up and purchase their drinking water. However, the water shops essentially have a carbon filter and a reverse osmosis setup, without adding back in any essential minerals. To me it is somewhat worrisome that this is allowed to be sold as potable water. Yes, it takes out chlorine, ammonia, fluoride and other toxins, but it also ends up being demineralized water. Drinking distilled or demineralized water is bad for you, so even in your house you would need to have a system that adds essential minerals and electrolytes back in, which is yet another expense.

Beside the long term health effect of the toxins and the killing of the good gut bacteria, I even noticed a burning sensation in my esophagus from tap water in California. This was the case even when using an expensive carbon filter. Now I no longer dare using unfiltered tap water even for washing vegetables. For drinking water I am paying a lot of money to have five gallon glass bottles of water delivered. In the shower I have installed a filter to avoid breathing in the chlorine fumes during bathing. If you start thinking about it all it is maddening.

The unhealthy tap water quality was yet another piece in the puzzle of my health issues and an inhibitor in my healing process.

As soon as I started using bottled mineral water I immediately noticed the resolution of a long term issue of a slight burning sensation in the esophagus. Over time I had fewer stomach and food sensitivity issues, better microbiome balance, and more energy. Of course water was only one piece in helping accomplish this healing, but it needed addressing.

Microbiome Dysbiosis

Microbiome dysbiosis, where the balance of good and bad bacteria is off, was established in my situation with a variety of tests. It included issues like SIBO, Candida yeast overgrowth, acid reflux, inflammation of the stomach and intestines, vitamin deficiencies, lactose and gluten sensitivities, impaired nutrient absorption, and neurotransmitter issues.

There is a good chance that if you have been enjoying the standard Western diet and chlorinated tap water, or are suffering from (pre-) EPI, CFS or a variety of other illnesses and symptoms, that your microbiome is not in balance.

Of course, being able to avoid getting ill from a pathogenic bacteria or heal from an infection is vital, but we went overboard in recent decades with the fear of all bacteria. So much so that most people automatically associate bacteria with something bad that needs to be completely eradicated. We carry more bacterial DNA than human DNA in the body; it is a symbiotic relationship. It is more important than we may think, to have the right amount of beneficial bacterial in the right place, and not too much of the dysbiotic bacteria or fungi.

There are so many factors that can cause this imbalance. It can even begin as early as pre-birth when the mother, if she has an imbalanced microbiome, can pass this imbalance to the child during birth. A natural birth instead of a Caesarian section, or breastfeeding, can help provide important bacterial baselines to the child. Over the years, poor diet, excessive sugar, artificial sugars, preservatives and other food chemicals, antibiotics treatments, chlorinated tap water, excessive glyphosate exposure, antimicrobial soaps and products, and household chemicals can all help cause a bacterial imbalance. Beneficial bacteria such as Lactobacillus, Enterococcus and Bifidobacterium are particularly susceptible to glyphosate. Those good bacteria were very low in my stool test, with Enterococcus too low to even be measured. Clostridium and Salmonella are highly resistant to glyphosate and showed positive in my blood and urine tests. Killing off beneficial bacteria often leaves space for detrimental dysbiotic bacteria and resistant ones to grow.

It is a medical research area that is recently, and encouragingly so, getting more attention. Microbiome dysbiosis is linked to a wide range of health issues, including inflammation, malabsorption, nutrient deficiencies, obesity, diabetes, autoimmune issues, allergies and sensitivities, intestinal disorders, asthma, cardiovascular disease, metabolic syndrome, neurotransmitter issues, mental disorders, anxiety, anger flashes, depression, immunity issues, hormone issues, and even cancer.

Microbiome dysbiosis causes a vicious cycle, affecting everyone of course, but in the context of those suffering with (pre-) EPI or CFS even more so. It hampers healing, impairs nutrient production and absorption, causes more oxidative stress and thus exacerbates pancreatic damage. Here are just a few simple examples of how beneficial bacteria can help us on a daily basis:

• Lactobacillus Acidophilus and Bulgaricus help digest lactose sugars in dairy products. Bifidobacterium and Streptococcus Thermophilus all use lactose as fuel and can help with lactose intolerance. This is especially useful when our inbuilt enzyme no longer functions well, or at all.

• Lactobacillus and Bifidobacterium bacteria help break down phytates, which otherwise chelate important minerals from the body. Phytates are often mentioned by the paleo community as a key antinutrient and a reason to avoid wheat and legumes.

• Lactobacillus and Bifidobacterium bacteria help with gluten break down and digestion. Is it not strange that there are so many wheat sensitive people these days?

• Bifidobacterium produces folate (Vitamin B9), which is needed in activities such as methylation. Both vitamin B9 deficiency and methylation issues showed on my tests.

• Lactobacillus Acidophilus can produce digestive enzymes like amylase. Those with EPI, where production of pancreatic enzymes is impaired, could certainly use the help.

• Beneficial bacteria reduce inflammatory cytokines, and suppress bacterial and yeast overgrowth in the small intestine. They also help with avoiding intestinal permeability (leaky gut) and inflammatory bowel diseases. Tryptophan also plays a role here.

• Oxalobacter Formigenes bacteria help metabolize oxalates in the gut. Oxalates are present in many foods from carrots and beets to almonds and amaranth.

• Most of the body's serotonin is produced in the gastrointestinal tract, with tryptophan as a key ingredient. Still under-researched, but I read that there are certain microbiome species which help stimulate the intestinal endocrine cells to produce serotonin.

• Melatonin production can be impacted because it is derived from serotonin.

• There are a number of tryptophan metabolites produced by gut bacteria, such as indole and tryptamine which are important in microbial composition and metabolism, the immune system, and intestinal inflammation subsidence.

Noise in the System

Sadly, the way big businesses operate along with willing law makers, makes it even harder to figure out the root cause of a health issue through all the noise. When industries help write laws, bribe (sorry, lobby) those that implement those laws, sue anyone in their path, manipulate the way research is done, and skew research for marketing purposes, greed wins and public health loses. Many non-profit and pseudo-health organizations, often with very highly paid executives, are complicit in unhealthy messaging. It is an incestuous relationship between funding and research by the same companies that help perpetuate the problem. Add in another set of companies that sell high priced patented pills which attack symptoms and do not resolve root causes. If millions of people were told they could prevent diabetes in the first place by following a few simple steps, or even potentially improve their type 2 with a primal or ketogenic diet, it would not help profits and executive salaries and bonuses of those pseudo-health institutions and manufacturers.

Take research studies and summaries on research studies you read in the news with a healthy dose of skepticism. A large portion of medical research is paid for by companies, and medical journals are then paid by those same companies to publish and republish only cherry-picked results. Peer review apparently cannot be considered as trustworthy any longer. Large percentages of studies never see the light of day, making it seem as if the effectiveness of certain products is more positive than reality. And so, the peer-reviewed, randomized, controlled, evidence-based research studies cannot be considered without some skepticism. It also makes you wonder how much sponsorship money as well as direct and indirect pressure is flowing into medical schools.

Just talk to your doctor about what supplements to take or what food to take or avoid in your situation, and you will likely get a very generic answer. Obviously there are many exceptions, and most doctors really want to help their patients. There are many who have seen the light, and are interested in continuously learning and adapting their treatments based on new information since medical school. Doctors that understand that the standard "healthy" ranges of lab results are not necessarily optimal for you, and who understand the potential positive impact of supplementation treatment. I would take the anecdotal findings and results from a doctor with their actual patients very seriously, even if not backed by an "official" double-blind research study. Luckily, many such doctors are sharing their knowledge with patients, online through blogs, and books.

But, doctors are often tied to a system which is forced to take on a high volume of patients with very short visit times, and thus have little time to really delve into root cause analysis. They are hampered by pressures from insurance and pharmaceutical companies, medical and pseudo-medical institutions, legal threats, mountains of paperwork and red tape, political correctness, social pressures and debt burdens. The litigious culture can hamper doctors from thinking about the best treatment for the patient, as they have to consider "CYA" maneuvers, insurance red tape and decisions, and time consuming administration.

Pharmaceutical companies are allowed to market directly to consumers on television and radio in certain countries, causing additional noise and pressure. I cannot remember how many times I have had to wait in a doctor's office whilst a pharmaceutical sales representative was monopolizing the doctor's time with their song and dance. Meanwhile, doctors have to be very careful in how they word suggestions regarding lifestyle choices, alternative treatments, nutritional or supplement advice.

Granted, for acute or standard issues there is no better than Western medicine, and pharmaceutical companies have developed many incredible, life-saving medicines for a wide variety of diseases. But for illness prevention, anything chronic or difficult to diagnose, you usually end up with symptom suppression rather than root-cause healing. Why do you think alternative medicine is such a fast growing industry? Clearly there is a gap.

CHAPTER FOUR

Tests and Diagnosis

Since pancreatic damage is so difficult to diagnose until it is often much too late, this chapter provides you with a detailed list of tests to consider and ask your doctor about.

Tests include key pancreas related ones, some you may not have considered before. Also listed are some preventative maintenance ones, and tests for pancreas related health issues such as SIBO, Candida yeast overgrowth, chronic fatigue, nutritional deficiencies, toxins, hormones, and sensitivities.

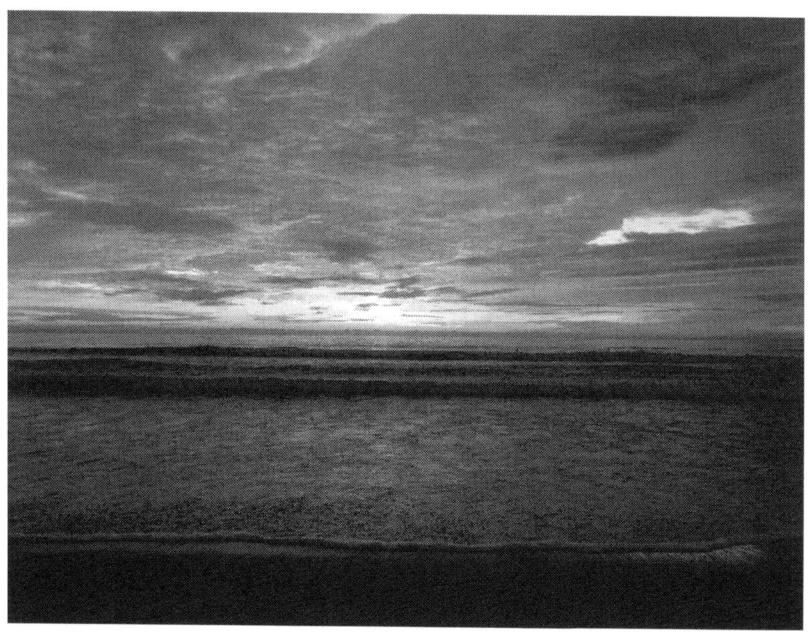

Of all the hundreds of tests I went through, only four were effective in helping determine the issue with my pancreas. Below I have highlighted the four I did as well as one additional one I did not do, but should be on your radar. If you suspect any pancreas issues such as EPI, have chronic or unexplained ailments, sharp muscle weight loss, maldigestion, malabsorption, malnutrition or intestinal issues, these are tests to discuss with your doctor. In this chapter I also share additional tests which might be helpful in analyzing your situation as they did for me. These include downstream effects of pancreatic damage, nutrient deficiencies, Chronic Fatigue Syndrome related issues and preventative maintenance. Additionally, I have listed some caveats as I discovered some tests are just not that useful, and a list of laboratories I have used, as some tests are very lab specific.

Issues with Current EPI Testing

Here is the sad and somewhat dangerous state of affairs when it comes to exocrine pancreatic damage testing and diagnosis. It is very difficult to determine whether you have pre-EPI or full-blown exocrine pancreatic insufficiency (EPI) until it is often much too late, and you are suffering from the consequences. EPI is usually diagnosed when over 90% of the exocrine function of the pancreas is lost. But does that mean you are not suffering and nutrient deficient if, for example, "only" 30% or 50% of the function is lost? No, of course not! This is what I have been referring to as pre-EPI.

Many doctors do not have the experience or knowledge to diagnose EPI or pre-EPI. On top of that, there is in my view currently a gap in the medical world to easily and cheaply be able to determine the specific level of pre-EPI. It would not surprise me at all if there are many people who suffer and die painfully without pancreatic damage ever being discovered as the root cause. A few issues to consider at this time:

1. Medical gap. A simple blood test to check for EPI or pre-EPI does not exist, unlike the endocrine side of the pancreas which is easy to test for diabetes and pre-diabetes. Furthermore, a simple non-invasive test to be able to discern at what percentage of normal you are producing enzymes such as amylase, protease and lipase in the pancreas is at this time unavailable. It would be extremely helpful and could prevent many lives from a slow and painful destruction. Accurate, standard, routine and early (pre-) EPI testing could possibly also be helpful for earlier pancreatic cancer diagnosis. Pre-EPI testing, when it becomes available, should really become a standard preventative maintenance activity for primary care or family practice doctors for an overall health check, not for just for possible cancer screening.

The OAT test listed below is the closest to a pre-EPI test I have found, albeit expensive. A blood test used by veterinarians to determine EPI in dogs should perhaps also be looked at as a potentially cheap and easy option; the immunoreactive trypsinogen (IRT) test. For humans it is currently only used if values are too high for e.g. cystic fibrosis, but is not considered sensitive enough yet to determine EPI or gradations of EPI. A fasted blood trypsin test is still worth doing to check for too low values. Perhaps in the future these tests could be improved upon.

2. MRI. Many people will likely not have their pancreas show up as atrophied as mine on an MRI if they can persuade their doctor to even order one. But, it is still a key test to do, as it can help rule out cancer and other illnesses. Pancreatic cancer is so deadly because it is often diagnosed too late, when it has already spread.

3. OAT as early warning. The amazing nutritional tests such as the organic acid tests (OAT) done by Great Plains and Genova Diagnostic laboratories are not on most doctors' radars. There is a lack of understanding on their importance and how to interpret them. They are essentially a practical application of biochemistry and the metabolic pathways' impact on the body. It is the single best test I encountered that can help as an early warning for pancreas damage, and as a way to get an overall preventative maintenance picture of your health. The reason for this is conceptually simple. Pancreas damage causes nutrient deficiencies, which causes metabolic pathways to not function properly, which in turn causes many metabolites and organic acid markers to show up out of range in the OAT test.

4. Amylase and lipase tests caveat. Important to note is that the two standard blood tests for amylase and lipase that doctors usually go for are utterly useless in determining exocrine pancreatic insufficiency (EPI). They are likely a cause of many missed diagnoses of pancreas damage. I had four doctors tell me that my pancreas was fine mainly based on those two blood tests. They might be helpful briefly during an acute pancreatic infection or duct blockage, when those enzymes spill over into the bloodstream. But, if you are not making enough of these pancreatic enzymes in the first place, they will not show up elevated in the blood. Do not accept any conclusion from your doctor regarding the health of your pancreas if these are the only pancreas tests they have done. It could save your life!

5. Invasive tests. There are a number of expensive invasive techniques that specialized hospitals do, usually after EPI is suspected or diagnosed. There are risks involved with any invasive tests since the pancreas is such a sensitive organ. Not to mention the weak state of our bodies in being able to fight potential bacteria introduced during these tests. The main idea with these tests is to insert tubes into your stomach and duodenum and stimulate, collect, and quantify pancreatic secretions in the duodenum. Examples are endoscopic secretin stimulation testing, cholecystokinin (CCK) stimulation, intra-ductal secretin stimulation testing, or a combined CCK-secretin test. I avoided these after consultation with my gastroenterologists, as the risk in my case was not worth any potential additional information. But it is important to understand the role of the CCK and secretin hormones, and the availability of those tests.

- **CCK** (a.k.a. pancreozymin or cholecystokinin) is a hormone that is released by mucosal epithelial cells when partially digested proteins and fats are released into the first segment of the small intestine, the duodenum, from the stomach. This in turn triggers the pancreatic acinar cells to secrete digestive enzymes, and the gallbladder to release bile into the duodenum. It also influences the satiety feeling.

• **Secretin** is a hormone that stimulates pancreatic ductal cells to secrete bicarbonate into the duodenum to regulate the pH level, and it stimulates bile production in the liver. It is triggered by acid entering the duodenum from the stomach. Pancreatic enzymes are inactivated when pH drops below 5, so bicarbonate and water is released to increase the pH level in the duodenum. Stomach acid pH is normally between 1.5-3.5.

Crucial EPI Tests

Too little pancreatic enzymes and eventually you can end up unhealthy, diseased or dead. Those with ME/CFS are also an obvious group of people who could benefit from these tests. Hopefully with these tests you can catch it somewhere along the line of the decline in time to try to turn the ship around!

Please do not be discouraged by skeptical or uninformed doctors. Try to persuade your doctor to get these tests done as they cannot harm you, but they may save your life as they did mine. Don't be afraid to question and research what your doctor tells you. If you want a specific test done, and a doctor declines it or does not understand it, find another doctor. If the doctor starts hiding behind jargon or is condescending, run to another one. Luckily, most doctors who helped me were very honest when they did not know something and appreciated the research and preparation I had put in before the appointments. They were almost all super friendly and very willing to help. I have found that with a little research you are in a very good position to analyze the findings from these tests. You also have much more time to dig into your situation than any doctor ever has. Trust your own gut feeling and analysis as you are your own strongest advocate.

Just be careful that you understand what is covered by insurance, or you know up front what the cost is. Call your insurance before having blood drawn or an MRI done. This was a hard and expensive lesson to learn. Anyone who has had tests declined as being "experimental", or received an insane bill after the fact knows what I am talking about.

Test 1: MRI of the Abdomen with MRCP Sequence

This is one that you might have to persuade your doctor for, but was the most important one for me in spotting the advanced fatty atrophy of the pancreas. It also provides great information on liver, stomach, pancreas, pancreatic ducts, and intestines. EPI can impact biliary secretion (bile salts are also key in breaking down fats), and so this test checks the gallbladder and gallbladder ducts as well. Ask for the MRCP (Magnetic Resonance Cholangio-pancreatography) sequence with and without contrast for better detail. It is non-invasive, painless and easy to do, although it can be a bit claustrophobic when inside the MRI machine. Just keep your eyes closed and focus on your breathing when inside. What I read in studies is that it is just as good if not better than the invasive endoscopic ultrasound and the non-invasive, but exposed to radiation, CT scan.

Test 2: Nutritional Organic Acids Test (OAT)

It takes the science of biochemistry and the study of metabolic pathways to a practical, simple to do and relatively easy to understand level. In my case they showed all of the following issues even before EPI was officially diagnosed:

- Pancreatic enzyme issues.
- Malabsorption and dysbiosis.
- Mitochondrial dysfunction.
- Candida yeast overgrowth.
- Small intestinal bacterial overgrowth (SIBO).
- Nutrient deficiencies including vitamins, minerals, fatty acids, and amino acids.
- Neurotransmitter issues.
- Oxidative stress issues.

AMAZING! I cannot be enthusiastic enough about these tests.

This is one test that can also be helpful to anyone with ME/CFS, or any chronic or unexplained health issues. Even those that are not ill could benefit by using it as a preventative means. If there is ever a test that should be done regularly by your primary care physician as a check up on your health, and to prevent nasty diseases and breakdowns later on, this is the one.

There are slight differences between the two labs I have used, but both provided me with information without which I would not have survived the last few years. It is also a great way to track and fine tune elements during your healing process. For example, it allowed me to track the success of my SIBO and Candida treatments, as well as adjust supplement levels down or up based on the results. These are the ones I have done and still do occasionally:

- **The Great Plains Laboratory**

Nutritional and Metabolic Profile (OAT and Amino acids)

- **Genova Diagnostics**

NutrEval FMV or ONE (Optimal Nutritional Evaluation) FMV

The Genova test now has an add-on section on essential and metabolic fatty acids, which is a great way to see whether your diet is too high in omega-6 (some of which are inflammatory), or too low in omega-3 and -9 (anti-inflammatory), or has good levels of monounsaturated or saturated fat. It also provides two helpful indicators, "Need for Pancreatic Enzymes" and "Need for Probiotics" that are helpful to anyone with pancreatic damage or microbiome dysbiosis. The Genova test also provides some toxic metal and essential minerals levels. I prefer to do the plasma amino acids as I have read it is more accurate, but I have done both urine and blood versions.

Test 3: Comprehensive Stool Analysis with Elastase

Either of the following two tests provides a valuable picture of your intestinal health. I still do either one of them occasionally to make sure I am staying on track.

• **Doctor's Data**
Comprehensive Stool Analysis / Parasitology

• **Genova Diagnostics**
Comprehensive Digestive Stool Analysis 2.0 with Fecal Fat Distribution and Chymotrypsin Add-On.

One additional confirmation of EPI on this test is the pancreatic elastase element. This is an enzyme only produced by the human pancreas, and thus, even if you are taking pancreatic enzyme pills it should not affect the test. Even if elastase shows the slightest bit under the threshold value of 200 (µg/mL), consider taking pancreatic enzymes as well as performing further tests. During my worst months my elastase showed 194 (µg/mL). This test should not be the only one to determine whether you have EPI, as values can fluctuate at different snapshots in time.

Genova provides an optional add-on to check chymotrypsin level, which is a pancreatic enzyme that breaks down proteins and can be measured in the stool. Keep in mind that it is less accurate than elastase, but still good to consider.

Another good indicator of malabsorption which can point to EPI is the analysis of short chain fatty acids (SCFA) that these stool tests provide. Since your ability to break down fatty acids is hampered, this shows up as excess SCFA levels in your stool. This symptom should quickly be resolved when you are taking pancreatic enzyme replacements and are breaking down fatty acids for nutrition again.

Microbiome information is crucial and this is also a good test to see if there are any intestinal parasites or other dysbiosis issues hampering your health and healing ability. It checks whether you are low in beneficial bacteria and high in dysbiotic bacteria. Dysbiosis can cause nutrient deficiencies (e.g., B and K vitamins), create byproducts such as ammonia, amines, hydrogen sulfide and can cause inflammation and intestinal lining damage. These exacerbate nutrient deficiencies, and can cause autoimmune, irritable bowel, chronic fatigue, leaky gut, and food sensitivity (e.g., gluten or dairy) issues. It checks for pathogenic bacteria that can cause acute illnesses. It is also a good way to follow up over time, and see whether probiotics, prebiotics, PERT, and dietary adjustments are improving your intestinal health.

Test 4: 24 Hour Fecal Lipids

This standard test checks how much undigested fat is in your stool. To be even more accurate you can do a 72 hour collection, but I only did the 24 hour test. With EPI, the pancreas is not producing enough enzymes to break down fat properly, and thus lipids can be elevated in your stool. For some it will be easily noticeable in the stool as discussed before, but for others the level of lipase production might be slightly hampered. Please note that it does not have to be elevated much to be an indication of an issue. It will also not tell you if other pancreatic enzymes that break down proteins (Protease) and carbohydrates (Amylase) are sufficient.

You are supposed to eat 100 grams of fat during the days of the test, but when you are already suffering this will be tough to do. Just adjust the test result for a factor based on an estimate of the amount of fat grams you have consumed. In my case I estimated about 50 grams of fat, and even then one test result was almost double normal. Taking into consideration that I had only eaten half the expected fat, in my mind I was close to quadruple removed from normal levels. However, during some of my worst times and before the official diagnosis my result was slightly under the 7 grams per 24 hour threshold. It is why also performing the other tests outlined here will be beneficial, as this test alone will not be sufficient to diagnose EPI. It is a test to repeat throughout your recovery to check whether you are taking enough pancreatic enzymes during your meals.

Test 5: 13C Mixed Triglyceride (MTG) Breath Test

This is a non-invasive way to indirectly test pancreatic lipase activity, i.e., fat digestion in the duodenum. It takes 4-6 hours in a specialized facility. It is considered a bit more accurate than the elastase test for moderate EPI, but can be influenced by other medical issues that affect absorption, or even the speed at which you pass food. Since my doctor had already established EPI with the other tests, this one I did not do as it would have been superfluous. But, if the elastase test did not confirm it for you, it can be one to consider.

Additional Health Tests

The tests listed above are the must-haves for suspected EPI. Since those suffering from EPI or pre-EPI are affected so broadly in downstream health issues, it is important to remove as many toxic stresses to the body as possible, as well as resolve any nutrient deficiencies. There are many other tests I completed, from leaky gut, neurotransmitter issues, SIBO, Candida, metal and chemical toxins, hormones, inflammation, methylation, genetics, to other CFS related issues such as Lyme, Lyme co-infections, viruses, and bacterial infections. Below I have listed those that helped me with the overall health picture. Please keep in mind that many tests are expensive and insurance may not pay for them. I am listing them here, not in any order, just in case they can be of use in your quest for discovery and health.

1. Spectracell Laboratories Micronutrient

Perhaps a must-have test as well. It looks at micronutrient deficiencies in white blood cells, and this test spotted my vitamin K and zinc deficiencies. It is not a substitute for the nutritional organic acid test, but should be seen as additive since it looks at deficiencies from a different angle.

2. Commonwealth Diagnostics International Small Intestinal Bacterial Overgrowth (SIBO)

A simple breath test for both methane and hydrogen producing bacterial overgrowth.

3. DEXA Bone Density Scan

Depending on how long you have been nutrient deficient, especially in magnesium, calcium, hormones, vitamins D and K, a bone density scan can help determine how much impact it has had on your bone strength. Mine showed osteopenia far too premature for my age.

4. Calcium Panel

Due to common deficiencies in vitamins D, K, and magnesium, it is important to check calcium levels. This includes the following standard tests: calcium, albumin (for corrected calcium calculation), ionized calcium (bound to other minerals), parathyroid hormone PTH (helps regulate calcium, vitamin D, and phosphorus levels in the body), osteocalcin (vitamin K dependent calcium binding protein). Even a slight increase of calcium in the blood can cause negative symptoms including pain, heart rhythm issues and fatigue. These tests can also help track possible causes of bone density changes.

5. Great Plains Laboratory Toxic Environmental (GPL-TOX)

The test checks for toxicity levels in the body from non-metal sources such as organophosphate pesticides, phthalates, benzene, xylene, vinyl chloride, pyrethroid insecticides, acrylamide, perchlorate, diphenyl phosphate, ethylene oxide, and acrylonitrile. It also includes tiglylglycine, a marker for mitochondrial disorders.

6. Great Plains Laboratory Glyphosate

It tests glyphosate herbicide levels via urine. It was not available to me at the time and I am not sure how accurate it will be if glyphosate is accumulated in, for example, fat, tissue or bone.

7. Cyrex Laboratories
Intestinal Antigenic Permeability Screen

It measures intestinal permeability to large molecules (a.k.a. "leaky gut"), which can cause autoimmune reactions, inflammation, etc.

8. Xylose Absorption (D-Xylose)

It is an older and time consuming test that I did not do, but it may be of interest since it helps determine carbohydrate malabsorption. High blood levels and low urine levels could point to kidney issues, but low levels of blood and urine xylose indicate poor absorption. This could be related to various issues like EPI, but also SIBO, medicines, parasites, intestinal mucosa issues, etc.

9. Doctor's Data Toxic Metals or **Quest Diagnostics Heavy Metals Comprehensive Panel**

Tests that look for toxic metal levels in the body. It is another important toxic load to remove from the body, as it can hamper healing and damage the body further. Quest's test does not go as low in measuring levels, but will give an indication. First, do one unchallenged by a chelator. Be careful with chelating, as the chelating agent itself might make you feel ill. The release of toxic metals into your blood can cause issues as well. It also chelates necessary minerals, so you would need to supplement afterwards with key minerals. If chelating, do this with a very experienced doctor, and only when you feel strong enough to go through it. The DMSA chelator my doctor used made me sick for almost a week, with three days of kidney pain and urine stinking of rotten eggs; all apparently known side effects.

10. US Biotek Standard Food Panel IgG

A food sensitivities and allergies indicator test. Although this might help remove an obvious irritation and stressor for some of you, for me it did not show any sensitivity. At my worst times, however, my whole intestinal system was inflamed and I was sensitive to almost everything.

11. Detailed Testosterone and Estradiol Panel

This is worth checking as a baseline, as well as tracking improvements in the healing of your body through pancreatic enzyme replacement and dietary changes. Testosterone also impacts your bone density. Any standard lab like Quest Diagnostics or LabCorp in the USA can perform these. Be sure to include total, free, bio available testosterone, sex hormone binding globulin (SHBG), DHEA-S and estradiol.

12. Detailed Thyroid Panel

This key bodily function can be impacted due to nutrient deficiencies like (magnesium, vitamins B12 and D, iodine, zinc, selenium, iron, etc.). Any standard lab like Quest Diagnostics or LabCorp in the USA can perform these. Make sure to have all six of these done: free T4, free T3, reverse T3, TPOAb and TgAb antibodies (to exclude Hashimoto autoimmune), and TSH. The ratio of free T3 / reverse T3 can then be calculated. Uninformed doctors still just do TSH and T4, which shows that they do not understand the thyroid. There are many overlapping symptoms with EPI.

13. Precision Analytical Dutch Comprehensive Hormones Advanced Adrenal Assessment and **Sex Hormones and Metabolites**

Since adrenal fatigue is a logical result of nutrient deficiencies, not to mention the stress impact of being ill, this is worthwhile doing. It tracks elements like creatinine, cortisol, cortisone, cortisol metabolites, melatonin and DHEAS over a 24 hour period. It also tests a number of sex hormones like progesterone metabolism, androgen metabolism, and estrogen metabolites. This is a simple urine test that can be done with a kit at home.

14. Celiac Disease Comprehensive Panel

Worth doing to see if you have celiac disease. My doctor tested for HLA DQ2 and DQ8, deamidated gliadin IgA and IgG, endomysial and tissue transglutaminase (tTG) antibodies. Please note that a negative result does not mean you are not impacted by gluten, and thus wheat. With EPI your microbiome is likely affected, and you can have a tougher time digesting gluten due to lacking sufficient levels of good bacteria that help break it down.

15. Helicobacter Pylori IGG

Standard blood test for the bacteria (a.k.a. H. pylori or campylobacter pylori) that can cause gastritis and ulcers. If you have pain on an empty stomach, nausea, loss of appetite it might be worth checking for.

16. Genova Diagnostics Oxidative Stress 2.0

This test checks for glutathione and glutathione peroxidase in the blood. Some of these markers are included in the Genova ONE (Optimal Nutrition Evaluation) or NutrEval FMV tests. It essentially confirmed that my nutrient deficiencies were impacting the production of the crucial glutathione antioxidant.

17. Health Diagnostics and Research Institute Catecholamines in Platelets

This test checks for adrenal gland produced hormone levels. It confirmed that I had low serotonin, which can point to low tetrahydrobiopterin (BH4), needed to transform tryptophan into serotonin. BH4 requires tryptophan, vitamin B6 and zinc cofactors in sufficient levels. The test also showed issues with transforming dopamine into norepinephrine, which could indicate vitamin C or copper deficiencies.

18. Health Diagnostics and Research Institute Kryptopyrrole

A 24 hour urine test which checks for elevated levels of pyrroles. It is another oxidative stress and nutrient deficiency indicator. Pyrroles bind with vitamin B6 and zinc, and thus can highlight deficiencies in them, and subsequent tetrahydrobiopterin (BH4) and neurotransmitter issues.

19. Genova Tetrahydrobiopterin (BH4)

A urine test which checks for neopterin and biopterin levels. BH4 is a cofactor for the enzymes responsible for the production of monoamine neurotransmitters (epinephrine, norepinephrine, DOPA, serotonin), and as a cofactor in nitric oxide production. It can indicate nutrient deficiencies such as vitamin B6 and zinc, and its subsequent neurotransmitter effects such as depression. MTHFR A1298C mutation, chronic bacterial infections, oxidative stress, or aluminium overexposure can also impact BH4.

20. Diabetes Autoimmune Panel IAA, ICA, GAD-65, IA-2A

To check for autoimmune disorders impacting pancreas insulin producing cells. Blood tests for checking autoantibodies for Insulin (IAA), Islet Cell Cytoplasmic (ICA), Glutamic Acid Decarboxylase (GADA or GAD65), Insulinoma-Associated-antigen-2 (IA-2A), and Zinc Transporter-8 (ZnT8A).

21. LabCorp Candida Antibodies IgG, IgM, IgA, Candida Antigen and **Fungitell assay**

To check for fungal infections, and if they have become systemic.

22. Antiparietal Cell Antibody (APCA), Methylmalonic Acid (MMA), Intrinsic Factor Antibody (IFA) tests

Since vitamin B12 can be impacted by EPI, these tests check for other potential causes of B12 issues, such as autoimmune causes of gastritis and pernicious anemia.

23. Prothrombin Time (PT)

To test blood clotting time, which can be impacted by a vitamin K deficiency. Mine showed fine, although the Spectracell test and bruising issues indicated a vitamin K deficiency.

24. Sigmoidoscopy

An invasive test performed by a gastroenterologist, where a camera is stuck into your rectum to check a portion of the colon. It allows for photos and biopsies. It is a valuable test to rule out other illnesses, especially if you have been bleeding frequently. It was quite painful in my case due to the volume of gas they pumped in. It did not show much in my case when I was at my worst, except to my eyes an irritated lining and remnants of very yellow colored stool.

25. Endoscopy

An invasive test performed by a gastroenterologist, where a camera is stuck down your throat to check the esophagus, stomach, duodenum and a portion of the small intestine. It is a valuable test to rule out other illnesses. If your doctor does want to perform this test, make sure that the necessary photos, biopsies, and aspirate samples for cultures and pH values are done. It was an unpleasant experience for me as I woke up gagging and in panic during it. Even when I was at my worst, it did not show much. Although, when I look at the images now I see what looks like an irritated lining. However, especially for those that have had chronic esophagus and stomach pains, burning or acid reflux, this might be worth doing.

26. Immunoreactive Trypsinogen (IRT)

Trypsinogen is produced in the pancreas and activated in the small intestine to form the enzyme trypsin, which helps digest protein. It is a blood test usually done to rule out cystic fibrosis in newborn children, where a high level would indicate an issue. Interestingly, veterinarians use this test in dogs to check for exocrine pancreatic insufficiency (EPI), where a level that is too low in the blood would point to insufficient enzyme production by the pancreas, and potential EPI. This is not a common test performed on humans to test for EPI at this time, perhaps because the threshold levels and EPI links are not sensitive enough yet. A fasted blood trypsin test is easy and recommended.

27. Genetic Testing

I did a bunch of these more out of curiosity (for example MTHFR for methylation pathway issues), but it did not provide much practical or actionable information in my case. Two genes that might be of interest as a potential explanation, especially if you have non-alcoholic chronic pancreas inflammation issues, are SPINK1 (Serine Peptidase Inhibitor Kazal Type 1) and PRSS1 (Cationic trypsinogen) genes. It is also important to know that just because you have certain mutations, this does not mean they are turned on. Perhaps in the future there will be affordable, gene-tailored medicine for specific situations, but at this time this is one of the least practically useful of all the tests I have done.

Preventative Maintenance Tests

Since EPI has such a systemic influence on the body it is also important to baseline and track other elements, such as your blood sugar, vitamin D and triglycerides levels, in addition to the nutrient tests mentioned earlier. These tests are good trackers of improvements over time, or indicators of potential issues. Looking back, the elevated triglycerides, HbA1c and LDL, along with low HDL, were big warning flags many years prior to my health breakdown. Ignore them at your own peril even if just slightly outside healthy levels. They are good indicators of food quality intake, and are simple standard tests that can be done at most labs.

Something that is a bit disconcerting in my experience is that doctors can be a bit lackadaisical or even dismissive about certain lab result numbers, especially when it contains nutrient related labs. You will have to be your own advocate, and with the wealth of information at your fingertips these days, you can be much better informed. One issue is strict adherence to the wide range of what is considered "normal" on a lab result, as this is often the range for the whole population. But is a healthy result the same for a twenty year old versus an eighty year old? You could feel horrible when, for example, your thyroid hormone, testosterone or estradiol levels are at the low end of what is considered normal, because for *your* body you might function better when it is at the high end of that same range. For example, you could start losing bone density due to low testosterone, but still be considered "in the range".

In the end we are responsible for our own health. If, for example, your triglycerides are elevated by 50% for decades, you bet there will be consequences. If HbA1c is elevated by a couple of tenths of a percent for years on end, you can be sure that you are damaging your body. Just because a level is a little bit too high or too low, does not mean you should ignore it. See it as an urgent message from your body to help you make a correction and potentially avoid serious issues later down the line. I wish I had known all this information twenty years ago, as many corrections are simple with hindsight!

My opinion is that these tests should be part of a standard and routine checkup for everyone, including currently seemingly healthy people, in order to prevent really nasty health issues later. Preventative maintenance tests to consider are listed below and in no order of importance:

1. Nutritional Organic Acids Tests

Discussed above in the crucial EPI tests section, and one of the best preventative maintenance tests I have come across.

2. Quest Diagnostics Cardio IQ or **LabCorp VAP Cholesterol Profile**

Detailed lipids panels that also shows the size of the cholesterol particles. Total cholesterol is not all that meaningful except as a potential warning sign of inflammation in your body.

- Triglycerides-to-HDL ratio should be <=2. If your triglycerides are too high, lower your sugar and carb intake.

- HDL should be around 60-90 (mg/dL). If too low, increase things like fish oil. Ideal total cholesterol-to-HDL ratio is <3.5.

- Bigger, fluffier particles of LDL and HDL are better.

- High triglycerides can cause higher LDL levels.

- LDL are lipoproteins which are simply the transportation mechanism for cholesterol and triglycerides from the liver through the blood to where they are needed (cholesterol), or stored in fat cells (triglycerides). If your body is handling an excess of triglycerides for storage, it needs to create more LDL to transport the cholesterol as well. This is why excess sugar and alcohol are such a big influence on cholesterol.

- HDL are lipoproteins which are simply the reverse transportation mechanism of transporting excess cholesterol back to the liver for processing.

3. Hemoglobin A1c (HbA1c)

Great six-to-eight week average blood sugar level indicator. <5% is ideal, and 5.3% or higher means your sugar and carb intake is too high, and you are likely starting to damage your body. 5.7% is pre-diabetic and is causing damage. The C-peptide test is also worthwhile, to check for diabetes and insulin production.

4. Vitamin D (25-hydroxy or 25-OH)

Healthy levels are around 40-50 (ng/mL) instead of 30 or below, which is usually when doctors start to notice. Some people prefer even higher at 70, but I think that is going too far in the other direction. >100 and you are definitely doing damage. In addition, you have to be careful to keep track of calcium and vitamin K, since they are closely linked with vitamin D, osteopenia, and osteoporosis.

5. Iron, Ferritin, Total Iron Binding Capacity (TIBC)

Standard blood tests to keep track of a key mineral. Just tracking iron is insufficient in determining potential issues.

6. Insulin

Normal is <5 (uIU/mL), but ideal is 3 or less. Higher than 5 indicates too high a level of sugar and carb intake, insulin resistance, and you are on your way to diabetes.

7. Fasting Glucose

Usually part of the CMP blood test, but it is easy to do at home to really get a handle on food influence on your glucose, and thus insulin spikes and sensitivity. Buy a little pin prick DIY glucose measurement device for self-monitoring.

8. Comprehensive Metabolic Panel (CMP)

A standard test many doctors order, which provides a wealth of info on your health and can be helpful to track over time.

9. Complete Blood Count (CBC) with Differential

A standard test many doctors order, which provides a wealth of info on your health and can be helpful to track over time.

10. Homocysteine

Indicator of inflammation and a number of health risks, including cardiovascular, stroke, as well as B6, B9, B12, or methyl donor (e.g., betaine, serine) deficiencies. It is seen as a better indicator of heart and stroke risk than total cholesterol, and a good one to track over time. Healthy is between 7 to 9 (µmol/L).

11. Gamma-Glutamyl Transferase (GGT)

A standard blood test which can point to liver or bile duct disease. Also important is the link to glutathione antioxidant production, as excess GGT can cause glutathione depletion.

Chronic Fatigue Syndrome Tests

One of the life- and soul-sucking effects of EPI is ME/CFS, with chronic fatigue, pain and malaise that can last for many years. Since the symptoms are so wide ranging and touch upon many areas within the body, it is not a bad thing to rule out other serious diseases. Chronic Fatigue Syndrome (ME/CFS) can have many different causes, but in my case it was exocrine pancreatic damage and subsequent secondary mitochondrial dysfunction due to all the nutritional deficiencies. Pancreatic damage is regretfully not a well-known cause of ME/CFS at this time.

Below is a list of other blood tests that I did in my quest to figure out what was happening, and to rule out other possible causes of ME/CFS. The caveat with virus tests is that IgM antibodies can indicate a current infection, but IgG and IgA show past infections, which could have been decades ago. In addition, knowing is one thing but taking practical steps to feel better is a different challenge.

1. Lyme and related co-infection tests:

- Lyme Disease Panel HNK1 (CD57)
- Tick Borne Disease Panel
- Babesia Microti
- Bartonella PCR, IFA, ePCRx3
- Rickettsia
- Yersinia Enterocolitica
- Borrelia Myamotoi
- Ehrlichia Chaffeensis
- Anaplasma Phagocytophilum

2. Brucella bacteria

3. Mycoplasma pneumonia bacteria
4. Chlamydia pneumoniae and trachomatis bacteria
6. High-sensitivity C-reactive protein (hs-CRP)
7. Lipoprotein-associated phospholipase A2 (Lp-PLA2)
8. Antinuclear antibodies (ANA)
9. Erythrocyte sedimentation rate (SED rate)
10. Immunoglobulin subclass IgG4
11. Interleukin-6 (IL6)
12. Carcinoembryonic antigen (CEA)
13. Cancer antigen 19-9 (CA 19-9)
14. Rheumatoid factor
15. Acetylcholine receptor (AChR) antibody
16. T-Cell Activation, CD8 subsets
17. Prostaglandin D2
18. Parvovirus B19
19. Cytomegalovirus (CMV)
20. Epstein Barr virus (EBV or HHV4)
21. Herpes simplex virus (HSV1, HSV2)
22. Human herpes virus (HHV-6)
23. Human immunodeficiency virus (HIV)
24. Syphilis
25. Coxsackie virus group
26. Hepatitis A, B, C, D
27. Human T-lymphotropic virus (HTLV-I/II)
28. Varicella-Zoster virus
29. Q fever bacteria
30. Malaria virus
31. Cystic fibrosis (CF): Usually tested for with newborn babies. It is also a potential cause of EPI.

Limitations of Certain Tests

Not all the tests were accurate for my situation, so always be aware of your symptoms and how supplementation and medicine impact how you feel. In addition, some of the standard plasma or serum tests might not necessarily show an accurate picture, as it only shows what is flowing around in your blood at the point of drawing. Your body can cannibalize micronutrients from muscle, tissue and bone to keep things going as long as possible, which may provide a false reading in the blood by not showing a deficiency. A couple of examples from my experience:

1. Coenzyme Q (CoQ10)

None of the standard tests were able to pick up on my deficiency, and I have not been able to find one which indicates the levels within tissue and organs, where most of it is stored and used. Only the OAT test gave hints via various markers, such as 3-Hydroxy-3-Methylglutaric, that there was an issue. Trial and error with taking ubiquinol and ubiquinone versions at various levels confirmed my deficiency, and helped resolve my heart PVCs (premature ventricular contractions) and chest pains completely.

2. Vitamin K

The standard plasma test was not useful, but the Spectracell intracellular test did pick up my deficiency. The deficiency was confirmed by my symptoms of abnormal bruising.

3. Magnesium

Another example where none of the standard blood tests picked up on the deficiency, but the nutritional organic acid test did. A negative standard blood test is logical since your body will beg, borrow and steal magnesium, which shows in the blood, in order to keep the heart ticking. Positive and immediate effects of supplementation confirmed it for me. Osteopenia indicated that my bones had provided magnesium to keep things running.

4. A, B, C, E vitamins

These vitamins never showed deficiencies on standard blood tests for me. The nutritional organic acid tests, as well as my symptoms and impact of supplementation, showed a different picture of many of these vitamin deficiencies.

5. Zinc, Molybdenum

No standard test ever showed a deficiency, but the Spectracell intracellular and nutritional organic acid tests all showed deficiencies. Supplementation also confirmed this.

6. Amino Acids

Another key issue with EPI and nutritional deficiencies are insufficient amino acid absorption. No standard blood test showed a deficiency because my own muscle tissue provided the necessary source to stay alive, with large muscle weight losses an obvious result. Once again, the excellent nutritional organic acid tests all showed large deficiencies and issues.

Laboratories

These are some of the laboratories to consider, some providing very specific and helpful tests:

1. Genova Diagnostics USA:

https://www.gdx.net/

2. Genova Diagnostics Europe:

https://www.gdx.net/uk/

3. Great Plains Laboratory:

https://www.greatplainslaboratory.com/

4. Health Diagnostics and Research Institute:

http://www.hdri-usa.com/

5. Doctor's Data:

https://www.doctorsdata.com/

6. SpectraCell Laboratories:

https://www.spectracell.com/

7. LabCorp:

https://www.labcorp.com/

8. Quest Diagnostics:

https://www.questdiagnostics.com/home.html

9. Cyrex Laboratories:

https://www.cyrexlabs.com/

10. Commonwealth Diagnostics International:

http://www.commdx.com/

11. Dutch Precision Analytical:

https://dutchtest.com/

12. Galaxy Diagnostics:

https://www.galaxydx.com/

CHAPTER FIVE

Supplements

Information on supplements by area of concern, based on my trial and error experience and success. Elements covered include nutritional deficiencies, intestinal, antioxidant, methylation, neurotransmitters, microbiome, mitochondria and chronic fatigue support.

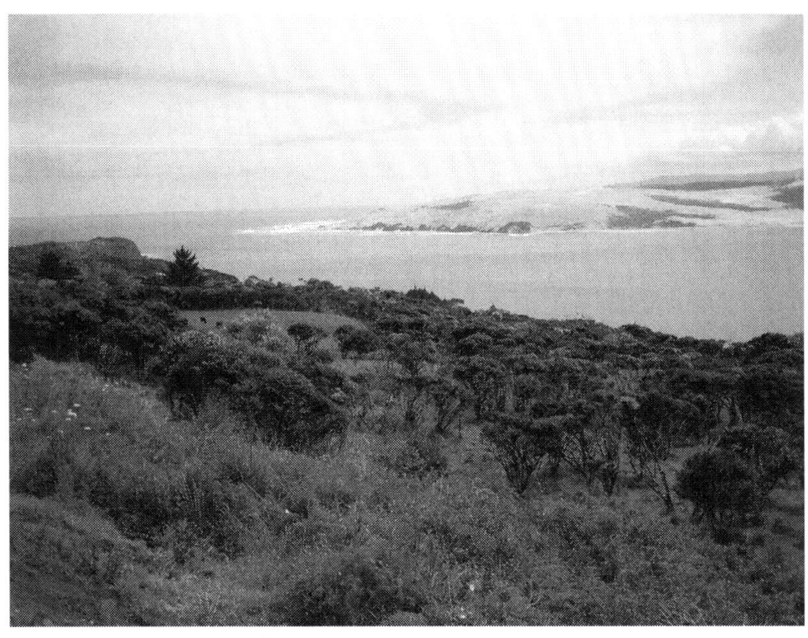

There are a few areas which may require specific supplementation attention for those with pancreas damage, especially for exocrine pancreatic insufficiency sufferers. This is needed to help heal and start functioning again. This chapter is split into a few key groupings that cover supplementation which helped me, not just with EPI, but also many of the downstream effects.

1. Deficiencies Rebalancing:

- Macronutrients
- Micronutrients
- Phytonutrients
- Fatty Acids
- Amino Acids

2. Mitochondrial, CFS Support

In this chapter, I have also included my supplements listing with details on type, brand and a description of how I used them. As a side item at the end of the chapter, I included a list of tools and home monitoring devices that helped me track certain health elements through these years.

3. Supplement Companies

4. My Supplements List

5. Home Monitoring Devices

In no way do I have any ties to any of these companies except for being a consumer, and I share them here to help you with a potential starting shortlist of items to consider.

Those suffering from pre- or full-blown exocrine pancreatic insufficiency (EPI), subsequent Chronic Fatigue Syndrome (CFS), or any illness or condition for that matter, will not have the energy to even start digging into the complex subject material of biochemistry and metabolic pathways. Therefore, I hope that the information I have gathered over the last few years will be able to provide you with some practical help, without having to become a metabolic medicine specialist.

If you are interested in more depth, there are many good sources of information on metabolic pathways and the impact of vitamins, minerals, fatty acids, and amino acids on the thousands of processes happening in our bodies, in order to stay alive and healthy. A few of these I have listed in the Appendix.

The nutritional and organic acid tests mentioned in the prior chapter are a good indicator of how well your body is doing in many of its metabolic pathways, and can help determine the supplementation needed to support your healing process.

Of course the supplements listed here pertain to my personal experience, but the process in which you determine which ones to consider is the same. It is a bit of trial and error since everyone's symptoms, bodies, deficiencies, and utilization will be slightly different. It takes time and constant adjusting of supplement types and dosages. So many internal processes that might not have functioned properly, or were blocked in some way, can slowly begin to function better again with nutrient rebalancing. The point at which to lower or stop certain supplements, because a health issue or deficiency has been remedied, is also personal and requires patience and experimentation.

Over time I have been able to really bring down the amount of pills I take per day. Keep in mind that too much of a supplement can also cause damage and undesirable symptoms. Once a deficiency is remedied, the recommended dietary allowances (RDA) listings are a good indication of what a healthy person would require daily. Certain supplements complement each other in in supporting a metabolic pathway, but others do not and should be taken separately. Some are better taken on an empty stomach, but other should be taken with food. Make sure that if you are on any medication that there is no contraindication with a supplement. Keep track of the quantities and ingredients especially if taking multis, as you may accidentally be taking a much higher dosage of a specific vitamin or mineral, as it can be duplicated across different pills. Supplement quality is also crucial as there can be a lot of chemical fillers, added sugar, poorly sourced ingredients, and even fake versions that will at best not do anything, but can actually cause issues.

One other action that I always did when finding out about a deficiency was to search for food items that were high in that particular micronutrient. For example, for magnesium deficiency I would add Brazil nuts, or for potassium I would buy some extra, not-too-ripe bananas. These days it is super easy to quickly look up a nutrient food list and order those items, no matter the season.

Deficiencies Support

Further in the chapter, I have provided a list of specific supplements that have helped me through the years to address deficiencies and imbalances. There are so many crucial vitamins and minerals that it would require a book by itself to go into the detailed workings of each.

With pancreatic enzyme replacement therapy you will be able to get a lot more nutrients from your food. After resolving additional nutrient absorbing issues like bacterial and yeast overgrowth films, you will indeed be able to absorb more micronutrients. However, depending on how long you have been deficient, deteriorating and cannibalizing micronutrients from your body, this will not be enough to replace the deficiencies initially. When you are suffering from pre-EPI or full blown EPI, you can have deficiencies in any or all of the following categories, which are very important in the healing process:

- **Macronutrients**
Calories for energy through carbohydrates, proteins, fats.

- **Micronutrients**
Vitamins, minerals, trace elements.

• **Phytonutrients**
Plant based chemicals such as carotenoids or flavonoids.

• **Fatty Acids**:
Essential omega-3, -6, and nonessential omega-9.

• **Amino Acids**:
Essential and nonessential building blocks of protein.

Macronutrients

Macronutrients are simply calories taken in through carbohydrate, fat and protein to fulfill our energy needs. It is one of the easier ones to supplement, but the key is to do it in a healthy manner. This means avoid anything non-organic, with added sugars, or chemicals of any kind. When you are taking pancreatic replacement enzymes you will now be better able to break down food and macronutrient supplements to actually absorb and use the calories, as opposed to just excreting them. Keep in mind that depending on the pancreatic damage you have, you still might not absorb as much as a healthy person would, potentially requiring a higher daily calorie intake. With EPI you will likely have lost muscle and bone weight. Find a high quality protein powder, preferably organic vegan or single ingredient whey, for essential amino acids and extra calories. I took a meal replacement medical food shake daily for about a year. Calculate your daily calorie requirement for your body composition. Also calculate your amino acids daily requirements. Especially the essential ones that your body cannot produce are necessary to be taken in daily in sufficient quantity. I used a Tanita scale for a rough indication of basal metabolic rate (BMR), which is the minimum amount of calories needed to keep the lights on. Until you are back in a normal weight range you can also add some healthy daily or multi-daily snacks like sugar-free nuts and seeds.

Micronutrients

Micronutrients are the vitamins, minerals and trace elements which you need to function. Trace elements are just minerals of which you need only a miniscule amount, hence "trace". The amounts needed of each micronutrient will be different based on your deficiencies, absorption and usage. Of course the ideal way to get these is through food, but especially in the initial healing period your body needs far more than you could possible get from your daily food intake. Over time you will be able to stop certain supplements and tone down others, as deficiencies are resolved and you are able to get the nutrients at the right levels from food again. But, four years into the healing process, I was still taking supplements in order to function better, albeit far fewer than before.

This is by no means an exhaustive or in depth listing, but I just want to share a few bits of interesting knowledge that I read in the many studies, websites, reports, books and articles during my experimentation with supplements during the healing period. They are not in any order of importance, but were eye openers for me. Depending on your personal test results for deficiencies, you might find different vitamins and minerals that require extra attention. The detailed list of vitamins and minerals that I took are in the My Supplements List section further in the chapter.

Antioxidants

Let me start with antioxidants, as I never really understood the value of them until I became ill. Now that I understand how oxidative stress, simplistically the rusting damage inside the body, was one of the key elements in getting sick, I cannot stress enough how key this is to supplement, especially during the healing period. Inadequate antioxidant function can cause mitochondrial damage and pancreas acinar cell atrophy. Realizing now the immense daily bombardment our antioxidant system has to process, it is amazing how long and hard it maintains homeostasis before finally breaking down in its weakest link.

Antioxidants can be seen as the cellular rubbish collectors which protect your cells from free radicals. A few key ones to look at:

• **Vitamin C.** For a long time I took three grams per day spread across the day, after my stomach was strong enough to handle it. One doctor suggested increasing the amount until I started getting stool issues, and then decreasing it back a bit as a way to find the right amount for temporary antioxidant support. I did not take it quite that far, and now I just sporadically take a little extra on top of a daily multi.

• **Vitamins A and E, CoQ10, beta carotene** are fat-soluble, so there is a good chance of a deficiency.

• **Alpha-lipoic acid (ALA)** is a powerful antioxidant which helps in, for example, cell signaling, damage repair and protection, energy production, insulin signaling, and the catabolism of keto acids and amino acids. It interacts with vitamin C and glutathione. This is usually present in multi-vitamin or mitochondrial support supplements.

• **Glutathione** is composed of cysteine, glutamine and glycine amino acids, and plays a key role in antioxidant activity and detoxification. In addition, there are a number of cofactors required in the production of glutathione such as selenium, zinc, magnesium, iron and copper, vitamins C, E, B1, B2, B6, B9, and alpha lipoic acid. Any deficiency in cofactors or amino acids can cause a decrease in glutathione. You can get a liposomal glutathione supplement, which you keep in the fridge and take a teaspoon of per day. You can also get vitamin supplement injections with glutathione in it. Both the injection and oral glutathione gave me cracking headaches, so I was not able to tolerate them. But, it might be worth a try to see if you are tolerant. If you are sensitive to MSG, which contains glutamate, one of the building blocks of glutathione, you could get headaches from glutathione supplements. Instead I focused on making sure the amino acid building blocks and cofactors were supplemented sufficiently, so that I could increase the levels endogenously.

• **Superoxide Dismutase** (SOD) is a key antioxidant enzyme which is tough to supplement. Supporting the process within your body, by checking your levels and supplementing any deficiencies in the necessary cofactors, such as iron, manganese, copper and zinc, and adding products like wheat sprout extract can help here. There is a product which has a bit of SOD/gliadin in it that I used sporadically.

Fat-Soluble Micronutrients

Because EPI sufferers have a difficult time breaking down fat, this can cause absorption issues and subsequent deficiencies of the fat-soluble vitamins A, D, E, and K, the carotenoid beta-carotene, and the often overlooked coenzyme CoQ10.

• **Vitamin A** is an important antioxidant. One noticeable symptom that it resolved for me was night blindness, and it also helped with blurry eyesight. Beta-carotene is a carotenoid, and a precursor which your body will use to make vitamin A.

• **Vitamin D** is crucial in many areas, from calcium and phosphate metabolism, cell growth, immune system, neuromuscular functions, inflammation reduction, to neurotransmitter production, and possibly glutathione production. Be careful not to increase your blood calcium levels when supplementing. Check your vitamins D, K, and calcium levels before and during, in order to fine tune supplementation. Up to 1000-2000 IU per day should not be an issue, however, especially when you have a vitamin K deficiency, it should be taken together with vitamin K. I notice more achiness if I take too much. It is also important in absorbing phosphates in the intestines. A very quick noticeable impact was improvement in my mood and wound healing. Testosterone levels improved as well. Fish oil also provides a little bit of vitamin D, along with omegas. Sunshine, without overdoing it by burning, is of course ideal. The ultraviolet B light will bind with cholesterol in the skin to help produce vitamin D in the body.

- **Vitamin E** is an important antioxidant which affects cell signaling and helps with mitochondrial dysfunction. Effects of deficiencies can take many years to show. It can interfere with vitamin K since it shares many metabolic pathways, so if you are taking vitamin K, keep an eye on your vitamin E intake. None of my tests showed an issue, but I still take it as part of a multi-vitamin. In the initial month after the diagnosis I took additional vitamin E each day.

- **Vitamin K** deficiency causes excessive bruising, impaired bone density, increased risk of calcification of arteries especially when taking vitamin D supplements, since vitamin D assists in absorbing calcium. It is needed to form osteocalcin, a marker for bone formation process, but it is also used in testosterone and insulin processes. My most noticeable symptom resolution when taking vitamin K was that I no longer had excessive and easy bruising.

- **CoQ10** is also referred to as ubiquinol (reduced form) or ubiquinone (oxidized form). Either form your body can synthesize back and forth, hence it is not a vitamin. But this synthesis does require methylation, so if you have any methylation issues, supplementation can help too. It is a powerful antioxidant that is contained in cell membranes of nearly all cells, but concentrated in high use areas such as the pancreas, heart, liver, muscles and kidneys. It is crucial in energy production through the oxidative phosphorylation mitochondrial function. Deficiencies have been tied to oxidative stress, diabetes, cancer, heart failure, heart arrhythmias, and neurological issues. This really was a miracle supplement for me, and after years of deficiencies my stores were clearly depleted. It had an impact on chest pains and heart issues, such as premature ventricular contractions, skips and stops. It was one element of the mitochondrial cocktail of supplements which resolved my heart issues within a week! This is one to consider for anyone with CFS, heart issues, taking statins, mitochondrial dysfunction, and energy issues. It took me months of 600 mg per day to start filling the storages again, before I could bring it down to now 100 mg sporadically. If I am low now, I notice a slight heart rhythm change or pancreas area pain.

Phytonutrients

Phytonutrients are plant based chemicals like carotenoids, flavonoids, resveratrol, and cannabinoids. They are important for your health and have, for example, antioxidant properties. Again, the best way to take them in is through as many different types of vegetables, seeds, nuts, and plants. As a supplement many are added in the various multi-vitamin or mitochondrial support pills. There are also many "superfood", "green" or "‘red" supplement powders that contain a variety of phytonutrients, and can be added to a protein shake. Just make sure you get organic versions sourced from trusted suppliers, without added sugar and chemicals. Some also add vitamins and minerals to the mix, so make sure you keep track of your total intake of micronutrients so as not to overdo it either.

Fatty Acids

Because EPI and pre-EPI sufferers have a difficult time breaking down fat, this causes impairment of absorption of essential and nonessential fatty acids, with subsequent deficiencies and health break downs. In addition, if you have been eating the standard modern Western diet, you will likely see an imbalance in omega-3 versus omega-6.

Fatty acids are absolutely crucial in a wide range of bodily functions, from growth and development, mitochondrial function, oxygen transport, energy generation, cardiovascular health, phospholipids synthesis, cell membranes, eyesight, neurological and cognitive functioning, to healing of wounds and infections.

Part of the Genova's FMV nutrition test I mentioned before shows details on your omega-3, -6 and -9 levels, saturated and monounsaturated fats, and interesting ratios to help assess health risks. The stool tests I mentioned provide feedback on undigested short chain fatty acids (SCFA) levels, which is another good health indicator and tracking mechanism. The main fatty acids are:

Saturated: There are a dozen different types, including omega-7, and are mostly found in animal products, coconut, macadamia nut or palm oils.

Monounsaturated: There are around a dozen different types including omega-9, which is a nonessential fatty acid found in, for example, peanut, almond, canola, or olive oil. Your body can synthesize it when needed, hence the nonessential label.

Polyunsaturated:

- Omega-3 such as eicosapentaenoic acid (EPA) and docosahexaenoic (DHA) are essential fatty acids found in, for example, cold water fish. Essential means that we cannot synthesize it and we must consume and absorb it.

- Alpha-linolenic acid (ALA) is also essential, and a precursor to omega-3. It is found in, for example, flaxseed, canola oil, walnut, and chia. The body can synthesize ALA into DHA and EPA, but only in limited quantities.

- Omega-6 is an essential polyunsaturated fatty acid of which there are around a dozen different types, including linoleic acid. It is found in, for example, nuts, seeds, "vegetable" oils like soy and canola, grains, hemp, most grains-fed meat and dairy.

NOTE: When you see trans (transformed) fats, interesterified fats or the very common hydrogenated fats on a label, avoid them as much as you can, as they are simply bad for you.

The fatty acid supplementations I have taken are:

Fish oil: There was only one over the counter pill that I found which did not cause those disgusting fish burps, and I experimented with dosage and duration. There is also a prescription version which only contains EPA and no DHA, with no nasty burps either. It also helps raise ALP, which in my case was too low. When you are able to tolerate it again, it might be preferable to eat a can of sardines or some smoked salmon during the week instead of a pill.

Coconut oil: Just make sure it is organic, in glass bottles, and without chemical junk. I used it daily during the SIBO and yeast overgrowth treatments, as well as sporadically for extra calories during healing times. It is also called MCT or medium-chain triglycerides, and is an easily digestible fat.

Olive oil: Extra virgin cold pressed oil in glass bottles, not pill format. Not really a supplement, but I was generous with using it in salads, on top of soup and in cooking.

Just be careful not to overdo it, as it can affect your cholesterol levels. Fish oil for example can raise LDL levels. Specifically the DHA component in fish oil increases LDL cholesterol, whereas the EPA component will slightly decrease LDL. Both EPA and DHA decrease triglycerides. Too much saturated fat and your liver can become overworked. In one of my experiments, when taking three grams of fish oil per day for four months, my LDL cholesterol increased by 21%, HDL levels increased by 11% and triglycerides decreased by 10%. Please keep in mind that taking three grams of fish oil per day is equivalent to eating one pound (454 grams) of fish per day! Too much olive oil will also show up on the OAT test, as happened during one of my experiments.

You can track your intake, under- or over-consumption, using the Genova nutritional test I mentioned before. Fat is healthy, except for trans-fat, and it is essential for the proper functioning of your body and healing, just don't go to extremes; all in moderation.

After my deficiencies were resolved and I was breaking down food again with the use of the pancreatic enzyme replacement pills, this was an area that was easily handled through food alone. Once in a while I still take a fish oil pill, but only if I have not eaten fish in a week. Olive oil intake is still daily as part of food and cooking. Coconut I have occasionally as a treat, but as the fruit rather than the oil.

Amino Acids

Amino acids, the building blocks of protein, are your friend. I had been trying many supplements and was on pancreatic enzymes for over a year before I stumbled across amino acid therapy. They are a crucial piece in the puzzle and something I had to educate myself on. A common misunderstanding is that to get all your amino acids you just need to eat more meat. What I did not know is that we, and the animals we eat, are unable to produce the nine *essential* amino acids. Only plants, fungus and bacteria can do this. These are phenylalanine, valine, threonine, tryptophan, methionine, leucine, isoleucine, lysine, and histidine. The other eleven are either semi-essential or nonessential ones that we can synthesize in the body if need be, and under the right conditions. Twenty amino acids are commonly mentioned, but selenocysteine and pyrrolysine are sometimes listed as well. Arginine, cysteine, glycine, glutamine, proline, and tyrosine are conditionally essential in the human diet, meaning their synthesis can be limited under certain health conditions, such as infants, illness or individuals in severe catabolic distress like those with EPI.

There are four big potential hits to amino acid intake and absorption to consider:

1. EPI or pre-EPI causes inadequate pancreatic enzymes to break down protein into amino acid components.

2. SIBO and yeast overgrowths hamper absorption.

3. Excess glyphosate exposure affects the metabolic pathway for plants used to produce the amino acids phenylalanine, tryptophan, and tyrosine, which can affect our intake. In addition it kills the good bacteria in our gut which help in the production of certain essential amino acids.

4. Chlorinated tap water kills our beneficial gut bacteria which help in the production of certain essential amino acids.

Amino acid supplements can be taken without needing to take enzymes, since they are already broken down from proteins. I was taking a multi-amino acid supplement, which includes all the twenty main amino acids, multiple times per day for many months. I am now down to just sporadically, since I am able to get it mostly through food along with PERT. The nutritional tests I had mentioned in Chapter 4 provide a great deal of information on potential amino acid deficiencies you might have. My body was actually using its own muscle tissue to fuel the requirement for amino acids in order to stay alive, resulting in a large muscle weight drop. The key to remember is that if you have an inadequate level of just one amino acid in a specific metabolic pathway, the pathway can suffer, with subsequent health impacts.

A good example is the production of the body's natural painkiller, endorphins, which requires many amino acids. If you are lacking in just one, the body has a difficult time producing enough, resulting in pain and lower tolerance to pain. Another area where amino acid supplementation can be helpful is depression. Tyrosine, tryptophan and phenylalanine, along with vitamins B2, B6, and copper are needed in the production of neurotransmitters.

Since it can be difficult to gain muscle weight, especially with EPI, consider taking an organic, vegan or single ingredient whey protein powder, or medical food to supplement with. You will need pancreatic enzyme pills when you take in a protein powder, in order to break the protein down into amino acids. This provides extra calories and essential amino acids. With a vegan option you will not have to worry if the cow from which the whey protein powder was produced had been ill or fed GMO, glyphosate and atrazine sprayed, nutrient deficient food. You are essentially cutting out a few middle steps in the process by taking a vegetarian or vegan protein powder. Mix up the types and check the amino acid contents for a good balance. Listen to how your body reacts to the different types to determine what works best.

There is a calculation based on the WHO chart below that can be used to determine how much of each essential amino acid is needed on a daily basis. You might need to take into consideration a buffer due to not absorbing it all effectively.

Daily Requirement of Indispensable Amino Acids from the World Health Organization (WHO)

Essential Amino Acids	mg per Kg of Body Weight	For 70Kg (154Lbs) Body Weight
Histidine	10	700
Isoleucine	20	1,400
Leucine	39	2,730
Lysine	30	2,100
Methionine (+ Cysteine)	15	1,050
Phenylalanine (+ Tyrosine)	25	1,750
Threonine	15	1,050
Tryptophan	4	280
Valine	26	1,820

Amino Acid Notes

Below are additional notes describing some of the functions of each amino acid, but is by no means an exhaustive list.

1	Alanine	Nonessential. It helps stabilize blood glucose levels.
2	Arginine	Conditionally essential. Used in immunity, insulin, cell division, wound healing and cardiovascular functions. It helps increase muscle and has a key role in nitric oxide production and cardiovascular health. It can help lower LDL cholesterol, but can cause bloating, abdominal pain and diarrhea if over- supplemented.

3	Asparagine	Nonessential. It helps brain function and has a key role in the synthesis of ammonia.
4	Aspartic acid	Nonessential. It helps in protective functions and detoxification of the liver, and participates in gluconeogenesis.
5	Cysteine	Conditionally essential. Cystine is the oxidized form of cysteine, which promotes tissue healing, is part of insulin, a source of sulfide, and a component of the antioxidant glutathione. Supplements are often in N-acetyl cysteine (NAC) form.
6	Glutamic acid	Nonessential. Important for neurological health, metabolism, neurotransmitter function and is a precursor to GABA.
7	Glutamine	Conditionally essential. Important for muscle tissue, neurological and gastrointestinal health, ammonia detoxification, supporting the immune system and glucogenic function. A precursor to glutamate needed to produce glutathione.
8	Glycine	Conditionally essential. Important in glucose balancing, formation of collagen, synthesis of creatine, growth hormone secretion, prostate health, nervous system functioning, bile acid metabolism, and key in glutathione antioxidant production
9	Histidine	Essential. Converts to histamine, necessary for inflammation and healing, is a vessel dilator and affects the central nervous system.
10	Isoleucine	Essential. A branched chain amino acid (BCAA) important for stamina and strength, recovery and repair, glucogenic and ketogenic functions, increasing anabolic hormones, and decreasing protein catabolism.

11	Leucine	Essential. A branched chain amino acid (BCAA) important for stamina and strength, recovery and repair, glucogenic and ketogenic functions, increasing anabolic hormones, and decreasing protein catabolism.
12	Lysine	Essential. Important for connective tissues, calcium homeostasis, fatty acid metabolism and may inhibit viruses.
13	Methionine	Essential. Prevents deposits and cohesion of fats in the liver, assists in gallbladder function, immune system function, methylation, blood vessel growth, creatine formation. It is a substrate for cysteine, taurine, SAM-e, and glutathione. High intake can increase homocysteine.
14	Phenylalanine	Essential. A precursor to tyrosine, epinephrine, norepinephrine, dopamine, melanin, and has been found useful in depression, lethargy and extreme mental fatigue.
15	Proline	Conditionally essential. Supports the immune system. It is found in collagen and cartilage, is important for maintaining healthy skin, cartilage, joints and repairing tissue.
16	Serine	Nonessential. Important in metabolism, linked to acinar cells, trypsin and chymotrypsin, a precursor to glycine, cysteine, tryptophan, and acetyl choline. Used in the transsulfuration metabolic pathway as a step in the production of glutathione, and it can help lower homocysteine. Linked to studies surrounding pancreas healing.

17	Threonine	Essential. A precursor to serine and glycine. Useful in certain neurological disorders, supports immune system, liver health, central nervous system function, and protects the digestive tract.
18	Tryptophan	Essential. A precursor to serotonin neurotransmitter, niacin, and the melatonin hormone. Related to stress reduction, sleep regulation and has antidepressant properties. Also used by good gut bacteria to synthesize components like indole or antioxidants. Uses the same pathway to the brain as the BCAAs.
19	Tyrosine	Conditionally essential. Important for catecholamine neurotransmitters, and helps with neurological balance, depression and memory deficiencies. A precursor to L-DOPA, dopamine, norepinephrine and epinephrine, as well as the thyroxine hormone from the thyroid gland, and growth hormone from the pituitary gland.
20	Valine	Essential. One of three branched chain amino acids (BCAA) important for stamina and strength, recovery and repair, glucogenic and ketogenic functions, increasing anabolic hormones, and decreasing protein catabolism.

The following are not official amino acids, but are often available or included as supplements in amino acid multis.

A	Taurine	Nonessential. It is an amino sulfonic acid, a by-product of the sulfurous amino acids cysteine and methionine. Important in cardiovascular function, antioxidant production, neurological health, anabolic process, mineral balancing, joint protection, bile acids formation, membrane stabilization, modulation of calcium signaling, development and function of skeletal muscle, and retina health. It is used in the transsulfuration pathway, can help in lowering LDL cholesterol, and can help with heart palpitations.
B	Ornithine	Nonessential. A non-proteinogenic amino acid synthesized from arginine that is important in the urea cycle. It is a precursor to citrulline, proline and glutamic acid. It is involved with insulin, human growth hormone, removing excess nitrogen and ammonia, and wound healing.

Mitochondrial, CFS Support

As mentioned earlier, mitochondria are essential organelles in animal and plant cells which are, simply put, the energy power plants of our cells. ATP (adenosine triphosphate) is the energy storage that they produce. They are in almost all our cells, and the heart, liver, pancreas, kidneys and muscles contain large amounts due to their high energy demand. Any dysfunction in the mitochondria can have a large impact on your health.

Due to the long term deficiencies, stress and insults to the body, your energy producing mechanism is possibly no longer functioning optimally. ATP production in cells needs to be supported as much as possible during the healing and recovery time, and beyond. One of my doctors had spoken with his colleague who specializes in mitochondrial dysfunction in children, and provided a simple mitochondrial cocktail to try:

- 400 mg of coenzyme CoQ10 per day.
- 100 mg of vitamin B1 per day.
- 5-10 grams of creatine spread over three times in the day.
- 3 grams of L-carnitine spread over three times in the day.

This resolved my heart issues in five days! I continued taking this combination for 4 months.

If you are interested in delving deeper into this area, look into the workings of the Krebs cycle (a.k.a. citric acid cycle or tricarboxylic acid cycle), oxidative phosphorylation (OxPhos), mitochondrial energy metabolism, or ATP. In the Appendix there are links to more information, including a great chart created by Genova Diagnostics (MetaMetrix) with an overview of the key points of the citric acid cycle. This chart shows the process from food intake to ATP generation, and the many steps and required cofactors in between. It provides a good overview of how oxygen, carbohydrates, fats and proteins are processed into energy, and at which points key cofactors such as vitamins and minerals, fatty acids and amino acids are required for proper functioning of this metabolic pathway. It provided me with an understanding of how easy things can go wrong, and how many elements are needed at the right time and quantity.

A combination of lowering oxidative stress and supporting your antioxidant system, as well as providing the cofactors needed in supporting your mitochondria in the production of ATP is important. The following supplements are worth considering for the energy production process:

- CoQ10: A fat-soluble antioxidant coenzyme. It is crucial and often overlooked, but it is hard to test for.
- L-carnitine: both acetyl-L-carnitine (can pass blood brain barrier) and L-carnitine versions of the amino acid.
- Creatine

- D-ribose. It is hard to test for, as it is quickly absorbed.
- Vitamins B1, B2, B3, B7, B9, B12, and E.
- Picolinated mineral complex: includes, for example, zinc, manganese and selenium.
- Zinc and copper in a 10-15-to-1 ratio.
- Magnesium
- MitoThera and ATP Fuel: Multiple ingredient pills focused on mitochondrial support.
- Amino acid support: A multi with all the essential and nonessential amino acids.
- Antioxidant support: Vitamins C, E, glutathione, alpha-lipoic acid, and Curcumax.

Other Notes on Nutrients

Below is a list of bullet points with additional interesting notes that I had stumbled upon regarding specific nutrients:

- Magnesium was an amazing supplement for me due to the many symptoms it helped resolve, and the speed with which it took effect. It helped with irritability, hypersensitivity to light and sound, pain, anxiety, panic attacks, sleep, asthma-like breathing issues, shortness of breath, paresthesia issues, blood pressure spikes, and heart skipping. I prefer the Epsom salt magnesium baths, ointments and sprays to get extra magnesium through the skin instead of through pills, but initially my deficiency was so bad I had to take supplement pills for months.

- Vitamin B6 is important for protein metabolism, growth, oxygen transport, blood sugar regulation, transforming homocysteine to methionine, and the nervous, endocrine, and immune systems. Absorption is complicated, involving phosphorylation and dephosphorylation, oxidation and reduction, amination and deamination, all primarily taking place in the jejunum and ileum portions of the small intestine. ALP, vitamins B2, B3, molybdenum, zinc and magnesium are all needed to absorb and utilize vitamin B6. B6 is also one of the cofactors required to synthesize CoQ10 in the body. Be careful taking vitamin B6 in large amounts as this can deplete magnesium levels and cause other issues. I will feel irritable and wired-but-tired if I take too much.

• Zinc, copper, magnesium or selenium deficiencies can lead to pancreas acinar cell degeneration. This reinforces the vicious cycle of pancreas damage.

• Important is a balanced copper-to-zinc ratio of between 0.7 and 1.0 in the blood. Do not just take zinc without knowing your copper levels and vice versa. Zinc lowers copper in the body, and when copper builds up it depletes vitamin C. Copper deficiency has an impact on mitochondria and ATP generation, but too much copper can impact your thyroid.

• Copper is important in metabolic pathways such as superoxide dismutase antioxidant production, dopamine, serotonin, norepinephrine, and energy production.

• Zinc, magnesium and calcium compete for absorption.

• When you take zinc, copper, magnesium or iron supplements, it is important to keep an eye on manganese levels. Manganese is important in areas such as digestion and metabolism, neurotransmitter production, antioxidant function, gluconeogenesis, urea cycle, cartilage and bone formation, and energy production.

• Manganese, zinc and copper are minerals which are all cofactors in the production and use of the crucial antioxidants superoxide dismutase (SOD) and glutathione.

• Molybdenum deficiency initially seemed strange until I found out that it helps detoxify byproducts of bacterial or candida yeast overgrowths. It is used in the transsulfuration metabolic pathway also known as the liver pathway, and is thus needed in taurine or glutathione synthesis. It binds to copper, so it can indirectly have an effect on the production of BH4. Certain genetic mutations can speed up the use of it, such as CBS, A360 or C699T.

• Low potassium is something I suffered from. One additional cause that I found out the hard way is that consumption of black licorice can lead to low potassium levels (hypokalemia). Licorice root contains glycyrrhizic acid which inhibits an enzyme in the body that can result in a drop in potassium, an increase in sodium level, and high blood pressure. This impacts the electrical signaling of the heart, and can cause heart issues such as palpitations and premature ventricular contractions. Low magnesium and low potassium often go together.

• Picolinic acid is produced from the amino acid tryptophan in the liver and kidneys, and is transported to the pancreas. It helps with absorption and transport of minerals in the body. During digestion, picolinic acid is secreted from the pancreas into the intestine. This process might be impaired with EPI, potentially impacting mineral absorption, which is why I added a picolinated minerals supplement.

• Vitamin and mineral injections to support EPI sufferers is something I interestingly stumbled on via veterinarians' websites, who seem to be further along in recognizing and handling EPI.

• Electrolyte imbalances are likely with EPI or any absorption issues, with subsequent health symptoms. Adding some high quality salt, or an electrolyte drink or pills can help. Just get one without added chemicals or (artificial) sugar. The major electrolytes are:

Sodium (Na)	Calcium (Ca)
Magnesium (Mg)	Phosphate (HPO4)
Potassium (K)	Bicarbonate (HCO3)
Chloride (Cl) Do not confuse it with chlorine, the disinfectant in tap water.	

• Important cofactors used in the transsulfuration metabolic pathway, which is key in methionine activation, homocysteine conversion and glutathione production are selenium, vitamins B2, B6, B9, B12, taurine, NAC (N-acetyl cysteine), glycine, and molybdenum.

• Choline is sometimes referred to as vitamin B4 and is derived from lecithin. Betaine is an important derivative of choline and in my case was important to supplement. Wheat germ, quinoa, grass-fed beef, liver, and eggs are all good food sources. Choline deficiency can lead to high homocysteine, which in turn is associated with higher risks in cardiovascular issues, osteoporosis and fatty liver. In my mind, just because it has not seemingly been studied as much, whenever I read fatty liver I immediately think fatty pancreas as well; the root cause is similar. Choline deficiency leads to deficient betaine (a.k.a. TMG, trimethyglycine), which is an important methyl donor and helps convert homocysteine to methionine. It is needed to synthesize phosphatidylcholine, a major component of cell membranes. Choline is also a precursor for the neurotransmitter acetylcholine, and impacts tyrosine related neurotransmitters like dopamine and norepinephrine.

• Serine, betaine, vitamins B6, B9 and B12 work together and are all linked to potentially lowering homocysteine levels.

• The importance of B vitamins in all the metabolic pathways are too many to mention, which is why it is key to get your levels tested and supplement them. Especially when first starting the healing process you can notice quick improvements with multi-B vitamin pills or injections.

• Vitamin B2 deficiency for me was exacerbated by my lactose intolerance and temporary gluten sensitivity. In the US, dairy and wheat products, both of which I avoided for a while in order to calm systemic inflammation, are fortified with added vitamins.

• Vitamin usages in the body are also linked, for example, B2 is needed for B6 to process amino acids. A deficiency anywhere in the chain can cause health issues.

• Cannabidiol (CBD) oil. This phytonutrient was a late one to try since it was not legal for a long time. I added a very small amount to help with chronic body ache and pain. I only used THC free ones, but there have been studies that mention a combination of CBD and THC helps with chronic pain. Since it is early days, the tough thing is to get trusted good quality that is without any cheap fillers or other toxins. I started getting migraine type headaches and dry-(cotton) mouth from CBD, so I only took a few drops per day for two weeks before stopping the experiment. However, many others have had great success with CBD so it is worth looking into.

• Instead of pills, especially when your stomach and intestines are really struggling and very sensitive, you could look into transdermal vitamin and mineral patches. I have not tried them since I found out about them too late, but they look intriguing as a way to bypass your intestinal tract to get some supplementation.

My Supplements List

Below is a list of supplements that I have used over the course of four years on my quest to feel better. Please keep in mind that this was based on trial and error, with my symptoms and my nutrient deficiency results on tests. Some I used sporadically, some temporarily until a specific deficiency was resolved, and others I still use. I have loosely categorized them as follows:

- Amino acids
- Antioxidant support
- EPI
- Intestinal healing
- Methylation
- Mitochondrial (also for CFS)
- Neurotransmitter
- Omega-3
- SIBO, Candida yeast overgrowth
- Vitamins and minerals

You have to be careful not to over-supplement as this can cause damage as well. Calculate the total intake for each vitamin or mineral especially if you are taking multi-vitamins and multi-minerals types of pills. Monitor your results with regular blood and nutrient tests, but especially how your body reacts.

My reason for sharing these is so that you have a starting point for ideas and brands to consider, as well as a brief explanation of why I used them.

#	Supplement	Notes
1	**Type**: Amino Acids **Supplement**: Amino Acids-All Basic Plus or Super Sports **Brand**: Montiff	For deficiencies, malabsorption, and catabolism. For a year 1-3 daily, 30 minutes before a meal or just before bed. Now sporadically.
2	**Type**: Amino Acids **Supplement**: L-Arginine Caps **Brand**: Life Extension	Once per day for 1-2 weeks to resolve a deficiency, and help increase nitric oxide, creatinine production, help with hypoglycemia and endothelial cell support.
3	**Type**: Amino Acids **Supplement**: Pure L-Serine **Brand**: Montiff	Sporadic. To help lower homocysteine and help with glycine synthesis. It is mentioned in studies of pancreas damage healing.
4	**Type**: Antioxidant Support **Supplement**: Alpha-Lipoic Acid (ALA) with Biotin **Brand**: Life Extension	Daily for 2 months, then sporadic.
5	**Type**: Antioxidant Support **Supplement**: Liposomal Glutathione **Brand**: Pure Encapsulations	For deficiency. Daily for 2 weeks, then sporadic. Intravenous drips with glutathione were tried as well. If sensitive to glutamate this may give you headaches. I prefer to supplement the cofactors and amino acids needed for internal production instead.

#	Supplement	Notes
6	**Type**: Antioxidant Support **Supplement**: Curcumax Pro **Brand**: Integrative Therapeutics	Initially 1-2 per day for about 1 month, then weekly for about 12 months. Can help with inflammation reduction.
7	**Type**: Antioxidant Support **Supplement**: Micellized Vitamin A **Brand**: Klaire Labs	1-2 drops per day for 3 months. Fat-soluble vitamin. Helped me with night blindness and blurry eyesight.
8	**Type**: Antioxidant Support **Supplement**: Nutri-E 400 Forte Vitamin E **Brand**: Douglas Laboratories	Briefly 400 IU daily for 1 month after diagnosis of EPI.
9	**Type**: Antioxidant Support **Supplement**: Endothelial Defense **Brand**: Life Extension	Contains superoxide dismutase gliadin complex as well as some phytonutrients. Used sporadically.
10	**Type**: Antioxidant Support **Supplement**: Super Ubiquinol CoQ10 **Brand**: Life Extension	For deficiency. Fat-soluble antioxidant that resolved my heart palpitations. For 1 month I took 600 mg, for 9 months I took 300 mg since I was so depleted. Part of the mitochondrial support cocktail. Now I still take 100 mg almost daily.
11	**Type**: EPI **Supplement**: Super Digestaway **Brand**: Solaray	Sporadically. It is in addition to prescription enzymes like Creon.

#	Supplement	Notes
12	**Type**: EPI **Supplement**: Creon pancrelipase (12,000, 24,000, 36,000 Lipase units) **Brand**: Abbvie	I take around 72,000-108,000 per meal and 24,000-36,000 per snack, depending on the fat contents and portion size. This keeps me alive.
13	**Type**: EPI **Supplement**: GI Sustain **Brand**: Metagenics	Medical food. Great way to get micronutrients and macro nutrients on a sensitive intestinal system. I took this daily for about a year or to get extra calories.
14	**Type**: Intestinal Healing **Supplement**: Dipan - 9 **Brand**: Thorne Research	If in an absolute bind with prescription enzymes, an over the counter version to take with each meal and snack. This is not a replacement for pancrelipase like Creon! I only took it before EPI was diagnosed.
15	**Type**: Intestinal Healing **Supplement**: Gl-Encap **Brand**: Thorne Research	Daily during SIBO and Candida treatment, and sporadic if my stomach is irritated. Contains deglycyrrhizinated licorice (DGL) root extract, marshmallow root extract, slippery elm bark, and aloe vera.
16	**Type**: Intestinal Healing **Supplement**: Glutagenics **Brand**: Metagenics	Daily during SIBO and Candida treatment, and sporadic if my stomach is irritated. Contains glutamine, deglycyrrhizinated licorice (DGL), and aloe gel.

#	Supplement	Notes
17	**Type**: Intestinal Healing **Supplement**: Pure L-Glutamine 500 mg 100 caps **Brand**: Pure Encapsulations	Sporadic to help with intestinal irritation and repair of mucosal lining. It is a precursor of glutamate, so if you get headaches from e.g., MSG keep this in mind.
18	**Type**: Intestinal Healing **Supplement**: Zantac75 or Ranitidine **Brand**: Zantac, generic	Only during acid reflux treatment. Divided in 3 times per day for 21 days maximum. This was to temporarily reduce acid and only in combination with other steps to calm the esophagus. This lowers your stomach acid, which normally is detrimental to your health.
19	**Type**: Methylation **Supplement**: SAMe (S-Adenosyl L-Methionine) **Brand**: ProThera	Methionine deficiency. Daily for 2 weeks, then sporadic. This is effective for depression, methyl donor, glutathione production, but can increase homocysteine. Combine with betaine for improved effect and less impact on homocysteine.
20	**Type**: Methylation **Supplement**: TMG - Trimethylglycine (Betaine) **Brand**: Life Extension	Sporadic. To lower homocysteine and provide a methyl donor. To help with choline deficiency. Mentioned in studies of pancreas damage healing. It seems to help me with pancreas type pain.
21	**Type**: Mitochondrial **Supplement**: Albuterol Sulfate inhaler **Brand**: Various	Only used during the months when I had real trouble breathing. This was no longer needed after magnesium supplementation and Creon prescription.

#	Supplement	Notes
22	**Type**: Mitochondrial **Supplement**: ATP Fuel **Brand**: Researched Nutritionals	For 6 months taken daily to help mitochondrial function. Since then, sporadic.
23	**Type**: Mitochondrial **Supplement**: Carnitall **Brand**: Jarrow	For 2 years taking 1-3 grams per day. Part of the mitochondrial support cocktail. Helped resolve my heart issues. Still take sporadically 1 gram per day.
24	**Type**: Mitochondrial **Supplement**: CorvalenM Ribose **Brand**: Douglas Lab	Took it daily for 3 months for mitochondrial support and energy improvements. You have to be careful if you feel blood pressure drops and dizziness.
25	**Type**: Mitochondrial **Supplement**: Creatine Monohydrate **Brand**: Jarrow - Creapure	Part of the mitochondrial support cocktail. 5-10g per day spread across the meals. The body breaks down creatine into creatinine. Took this daily for 6 months with my meals.
26	**Type**: Mitochondrial **Supplement**: MitoThera, MitoTone **Brand**: Prothera, Douglas Lab	Mitochondrial support with multiple ingredients. Took 2-4 pills daily for a year. Now sporadic.
27	**Type**: Mitochondrial **Supplement**: PQQ (Pyrroloquinoline Quinone disodium salt) **Brand**: Life Extension	Daily for 2 months. Mitochondrial support.

#	Supplement	Notes
28	**Type**: Mitochondrial **Supplement**: Phophaline Phosphatidylcholine **Brand**: Xymogen	Daily for 2 months. Mitochondrial support and an important component of lecithin. Important for cell membrane and oxidative stress repair, homocysteine regulation. Choline is sometimes called vitamin B4 and is essential.
29	**Type**: Mitochondrial **Supplement**: ResveraCel Nicotinamide Riboside, Betaine, Quercetin, Trans Resveratol, Niacell - Nicotinamide Riboside **Brand**: Thorne Research	Daily for 6 months. Mitochondrial support, DNA repair, inflammation support, insulin sensitivity, cholesterol and fatty acid synthesis support. Can help with lowering LDL. It is a precursor of NAD. Now take it sporadically around once every 2 weeks.
30	**Type**: Nausea **Supplement**: Ondansetron, Promethazine **Brand**: Various	Sporadic only during the worst of times for nausea in order to keep food down. Prescription only.
31	**Type**: Neurotransmitter **Supplement**: 5-HTP **Brand**: Ortho Molecular Products	5-Hydroxytryptophan. An essential amino acid needed to produce serotonin. Tryptophan can help with depression and mood. Sporadic use.
32	**Type**: Neurotransmitter **Supplement**: D,L-Phenylalanine. **Brand**: Life Extension	Essential amino acid. A precursor to tyrosine, which is needed to produce dopamine. Sporadic use for depression and mood.

#	Supplement	Notes
33	**Type**: Neurotransmitter **Supplement**: Dopa-Mind **Brand**: Life Extension	Wild green oat extract and calcium. Sporadic use to help with depression and mood.
34	**Type**: Neurotransmitter **Supplement**: Neuro-Balance (Tyrosine, B6) **Brand**: Montiff	Key precursors for dopamine to help with depression and mood. Daily for 3 months then sporadic. Be careful to calculate your total B6 intake.
35	**Type**: Neurotransmitter **Supplement**: Pure L-Tyrosine **Brand**: Montiff	Amino acid supplementation. It is needed to produce dopamine. Sporadic use to help with depression and mood.
36	**Type**: Omega-3 **Supplement**: EPA 120 gel Omega-3, Vascepa (prescription EPA only) **Brand**: Wiley's Peak, Amarin Pharmaceuticals	No nasty burps from these. 3 months 1-3 pills daily, then sporadic around once per week. Lowers triglycerides and provides important omega-3 fatty acids. Be careful as the DHA component raises LDL cholesterol and 3 gram fish oil is the equivalent of a pound of fish! Vascepa only contains EPA.
37	**Type**: SIBO, Candida yeast overgrowth **Supplement**: Biocidin Advanced Formula **Brand**: Bio-Botanical Research	Used only during the treatment of Candida (4 weeks) and SIBO (3 weeks) as it is a strong botanical microbial agent with many ingredients. 5 drops 3 times per day with a slow build up.

#	Supplement	Notes
38	**Type**: SIBO, Candida yeast overgrowth **Supplement**: Neomycin **Brand**: Prescription	10 days antibiotics course taken for SIBO. Taken together with Rifaximin (Xifaxan) for better results.
39	**Type**: SIBO, Candida yeast overgrowth **Supplement**: Interfase Plus Enzymes **Brand**: Klaire Labs	Used only during the treatment of Candida (4 weeks) and SIBO (3 weeks). This helps disrupt the biofilm of the bacteria and yeast. Important to take along with the other anti-SIBO and anti-Candida supplements, diet and medicine.
40	**Type**: SIBO, Candida yeast overgrowth **Supplement**: MCT oil from coconut **Brand**: Various	Used daily during the treatment of Candida (4 weeks) and SIBO (3 weeks). The caprylic acid in coconut oil is effective by penetrating the cell wall of yeast, causing it to rupture. After that sporadically as extra easily absorbed calories and fatty acids.
41	**Type**: SIBO, Candida yeast overgrowth **Supplement**: Molybdenum Chelated, Molybdenum Glycinate **Brand**: Thorne Research	To help with deficiency and Candida treatment. It is used in the body to break down a Candida by-product acetaldehyde (neurotoxin). Taken daily for 3 months, then sporadic.
42	**Type**: SIBO, Candida yeast overgrowth **Supplement**: Nystatin Antifungal **Brand**: Prescription	1 million units daily for 1 month for Candida overgrowth treatment. From a compounding pharmacy with doctor's prescription.

#	Supplement	Notes
43	**Type**: SIBO, Candida yeast overgrowth **Supplement**: Oregano SAP **Brand**: Various	Sporadic. To help microbiome rebalancing and anti-SIBO, anti-Candida effects. It is also an ingredient in Biocidin.
44	**Type**: SIBO, Candida yeast overgrowth **Supplement**: Probio Max DF, Probiotic Complete, Ther-Biotic Complete, Various **Brand**: Xymogen, Klaire Labs	Probiotics. Used multiple times per day, 30 minutes prior to a meal during SIBO and Candida treatments. Also used daily whenever on an antibiotic treatment. For microbiome dysbiosis, to help rebuild beneficial bacteria.
45	**Type**: SIBO, Candida yeast overgrowth **Supplement**: Saccharomycin DF **Brand**: Xymogen	Probiotic yeast Saccharomyces boulardii. Used daily during the treatment of Candida (4 weeks) and SIBO (3 weeks) for microbiome rebalancing.
46	**Type**: SIBO, Candida yeast overgrowth **Supplement**: Rifaximin **Brand**: Xifaxan	10 day antibiotics course taken for SIBO treatment. Should be taken together with Neomycin for better results.
47	**Type**: SIBO, Candida yeast overgrowth **Supplement**: Serralase - Proteolytic Enzyme Blend **Brand**: Prothera	Daily during the SIBO and Candida treatments. Contains bromelain, papain, catalase, peptidase enzymes. Helps break down biofilm. Sporadically afterwards to support tissue repair and maintenance.

#	Supplement	Notes
48	**Type**: Vitamins, Minerals **Supplement**: Active B12 - Folate (B9) **Brand**: ProThera	For deficiencies, malabsorption, and MTHFR support. Every other day for 3 months, then 1 every 1-3 weeks.
49	**Type**: Vitamins, Minerals **Supplement**: B complex - B Activ, B Complete, Stress B-Complex **Brand**: Xymogen, Montiff, Thorne	For deficiencies. Daily for 2 months, then 1 every 1-3 weeks for 6 months. Taken sporadically now when feeling extra tired.
50	**Type**: Vitamins, Minerals **Supplement**: B Complex Injection **Brand**: Various	For deficiencies and malabsorption. 4 shots a week apart to kick start healing. Careful not to overdo it. Make sure it has hydroxy or methyl, but not cyano version of B12.
51	**Type**: Vitamins, Minerals **Supplement**: Bone Restore with Vitamin K2, Osteocare, **Brand**: Life Extension, Vitabiotics	To help with deficiencies causing osteopenia and osteoporosis. Took daily for 1 month, then sporadically.
52	**Type**: Vitamins, Minerals **Supplement**: Buffered Vitamin C **Brand**: Integrative Therapeutics, Klaire Labs	Buffered with minerals to improve absorption, and avoid nausea and sensitivity issues. Important antioxidant. Taken 1-3 grams per day for 2 years, then 1 gram per day for a year. Now, sporadically.

#	Supplement	Notes
53	**Type**: Vitamins, Minerals **Supplement**: Copper (glycinate) **Brand**: Pure Encapsulations	Sporadic. Taken every other day 1 pill (2 g) together with Zinc for 2-3 months when I was deficient in both. I took 12-to-1 (Zinc-to-Copper) ratio in supplements. Copper deficiency has an impact on mitochondria and ATP.
54	**Type**: Vitamins, Minerals **Supplement**: Mag Complete, Magnesium Glycenate, Magnesium bis-Glycenate **Brand**: Complementary Prescriptions, Prothera, Metagenics	For deficiencies. Find one that does not upset your intestines. Some like liposomal versions. The citrate version is often used for constipation. Daily for 6 months with amazing results within days, then sporadic. To avoid intestinal irritation I use mostly ointment, mineral bath and oil versions now.
55	**Type**: Vitamins, Minerals **Supplement**: Magnesium, Vit D, Calcium **Brand**: ProThera	To help with deficiencies causing osteopenia and osteoporosis. Took daily for 1 month, then once per week for a year.
56	**Type**: Vitamins, Minerals **Supplement**: Multi Minerals: Mineral Complex, Pic-Mins picolinate minerals **Brand**: Montiff, Thorne Research	For deficiencies. Depending on other multi intake I alternated between brands. 1 every day or two for 1 year. Picolinic acid is a natural organic acid produced in the body by conversion of the amino acid tryptophan. This is likely impaired with EPI. Calculate total intake to not overdo it.

#	Supplement	Notes
57	**Type**: Vitamins, Minerals **Supplement**: Multi Vitamins: Vita-Minz Plus, PhytoMulti, MultiThera 1, A-Z Depot **Brand**: Montiff, Metagenics, Prothera, DoppelHerz	For deficiencies, malabsorption, and malnutrition. Depending on other mineral, multi-mineral or vitamin intake I alternate between the brands, but usually take one every 1-2 days. Calculate total individual nutrient intake to not overdo it.
58	**Type**: Vitamins, Minerals **Supplement**: Potassium Glycinate amino acid complex **Brand**: Solgar, Prescription	To resolve deficiencies and to help in resolving heart palpitations. Careful not to take too much at once. Taken daily for 2 weeks and then just sporadically or if I have a very rare licorice treat.
59	**Type**: Vitamins, Minerals **Supplement**: Super K **Brand**: Life Extension	Vitamins K1, K2-4, K2-7, C. For a few months, once every 1-3 weeks with vitamin D, after my K deficiency was resolved. Now sporadically.
60	**Type**: Vitamins, Minerals **Supplement**: Pure Epsom (magnesium) Salt Soaking Solution, Magnesium Epsom Salt Lotion, Magnesium Oil spray **Brand**: Dr. Teal, Morton, Various,	For inflammation, deficiency and an alternative method of absorbing magnesium without intestinal issues. Epsom salt hot baths also help with pain, anxiety and stress. For many months every 1-2 days. Ointment or oil sprays are good for topical application in specific locations, e.g., cramp in foot or pain in elbow.

#	Supplement	Notes
61	**Type**: Vitamins, Minerals **Supplement**: Tri-Phos-B **Brand**: Montiff	Vitamins B1, B2, and B6 for deficiencies. Taken daily for 3 months, then sporadic.
62	**Type**: Vitamins, Minerals **Supplement**: Vitamin B1 **Brand**: Various	Part of the mitochondrial support cocktail. 100 mg per day for 4 months.
63	**Type**: Vitamins, Minerals **Supplement**: Vitamin B2 **Brand**: Various	For deficiency. Daily for 2 months, but now sporadically around 100 mg weekly, especially when urine has a greenish tint.
64	**Type**: Vitamins, Minerals **Supplement**: Vitamin B6, P-5-P (Pyridoxal 5'-phosphate) **Brand**: Klaire Labs	For deficiencies. Daily for 2 months, then sporadic. Be careful not to take too much when adding up all the supplements that have B6.
65	**Type**: Vitamins, Minerals **Supplement**: Vitamin D3 **Brand**: Xymogen, Country Life	For deficiency and in support of bones, testosterone, immune system, insulin secretion to name a few. Daily 2000-5000 IU for 2 years. Now around 1000-2000 IU weekly. Careful not to overdo it, and watch vitamin K as well. Too much D and I get achy.

#	Supplement	Notes
66	**Type**: Vitamins, Minerals **Supplement**: Vitamin D3/K2 **Brand**: Douglas laboratories	For deficiency. Fat-soluble vitamin. Taken daily for 3 months to resolve K deficiency. Vitamin K is also important for vitamin D and calcium absorption.
67	**Type**: Vitamins, Minerals **Supplement**: Zicam - Zinc aceticum, gluconicum **Brand**: Zicam	Sporadic, only when feeling extra under the weather. Helps boost the immune system. Your body uses more zinc during extra immune system workloads.
68	**Type**: Vitamins, Minerals **Supplement**: Zinc Picolinate 25mg **Brand**: Cardiovascular Research	For immune system support, deficiency, and malabsorption. Almost daily 25 mg for a year. Be careful to calculate total intake, as it is often in multi-vitamins and multi-minerals pills. Zinc-to-copper ratio is also important.

Supplement Companies

Since it is hard to be sure of quality and origin of the ingredients in supplements, I use mostly the ones that were recommended by doctors. Of course there are many other quality brands, but these are just the ones I have experienced. Some of the basic vitamins and minerals I would get from commonly available brands in the supermarket, but please always read the ingredients for undesirable fillers, sugars or sourcing.

- Doppelherz (Queisser)
- Douglas Laboratories
- Integrative Therapeutics
- Jarrow
- Klaire Labs
- Life Extension
- Metagenics
- Montiff
- Ortho Molecular Products
- Prothera
- Pure Encapsulations
- Researched Nutritionals
- Thorne
- Xymogen

Home Monitoring Tools

There are a few handy tools and monitoring devices that you can purchase for home use. Of course there are many other good options available that perform similar duties.

Devices	Type	Note
Blood glucose or diabetes meter	Nipro Diagnostics TRUEtrack	Checks the impact of food and drinks on your blood sugar level. Learn how food, exercise, timing and glycemic index of food impact results. It is highly recommended to learn how your diet impacts your blood glucose level. I still use it quite often.
Blood pressure meter	Omron BP742N	Track changes and impact of diet and supplement changes over time.
Fingertip pulse oximeter	Acc U Rate Pro Series CMS 500DL	Heart rate and blood oxygen saturation monitor
Blood ketone and glucose meter	Keto Mojo TD-4279	Checks your ketone level in the blood. See how diet impacts fat burning versus sugar burning states. More accurate than urine strips.
Acid food and beverage testing tool	Dr. Meter 0.1pH High Accuracy pH Meter/Pen	Checks acidity of drinks during acid reflux diet.
Scale with body composition monitor	Tanita Inner Scan 50	Indicates weight, body fat %, body water %, muscle mass, metabolic age, bone mass, visceral fat, and basal metabolic rate.

Devices	Type	Note
Urine strips. Ten Parameter Urinalysis	Healthy Wiser	Rough check of urine with ten different parameters.
Urine strips. SEOH Indicator to detect sulfite or sulfate	Quantofix	Sulfite or sulfate dipsticks to check urine levels.
EMF (Electro-magnetic Field) meter	Trifield 100XE	Affordable, simple tool to check for EMF fields, e.g., where you sleep, work, and from any electronic gadgets.
Air filter	Philips 1000 series or BlueAir	Get one with at least a HEPA filter, but a real time sensor is also very helpful.
Air quality sensor	Temtop LKC-1000S	If your air filter does not have a sensor, this indicates air quality for PM2.5 and PM10 (µg/m3) particles, HCHO and TVOC.
Smart phone food tracker and calorie counting application	NetDiary App	Provides calorie break down, food tracking per meal, food database access and a barcode scanner.
Smartphone or pad meditation application	Headspace	Various time based guided meditations.

CHAPTER SIX

Food and Water

A significant underlying root cause of pancreatic damage should be addressed immediately in order to heal.

Food and water quality also happens to be the essential nurturing and healing element on the path to improving quality of life.

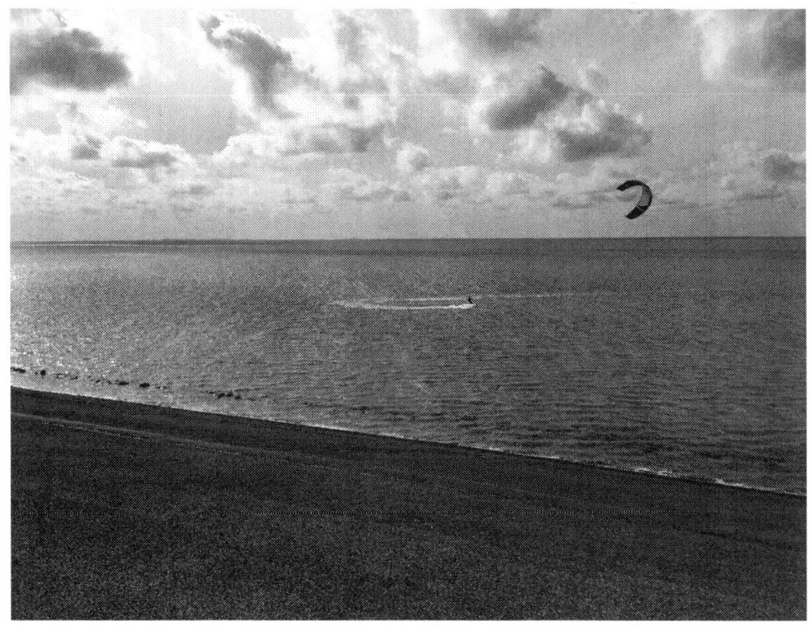

Metabolic Medicine

"Biochemistry and medicine are intimately related. Health depends on a harmonious balance of biochemical reactions occurring in the body, and disease reflects abnormalities in biomolecules, reactions, or processes."

Harper's Illustrated Biochemistry

Doctors often see biochemistry as a tough, long forgotten, university subject, and often do not receive much practical nutritional training. Exocrine pancreatic insufficiency (EPI) causes nutrient deficiencies, which in turn can cause hundreds of snowballing health effects due to no longer having this harmonious balance of biochemical reactions in the body. Metabolic pathways in our bodies can only function with, not only the consumption of, but the absorption of the essential daily vitamins, minerals, fatty acids, and amino acids.

Metabolic medicine should be its own specialty, working closely together with primary care physicians and any chronic disease specialists. It should be part of standard preventative maintenance healthcare, and the first line of defense in any chronic cases or those that are not easily explained. Biochemistry is basically how our bodies and their metabolic pathways function. Food and drink broken down really are just the carbohydrates, vitamins, minerals, amino acids, fatty acids, etc. used in these metabolic pathways of the body.

Food, water and supplementation play a crucial role in getting the metabolic pathways, and thus our bodies, functioning properly again. This is especially important for those battling illness, stress, pancreas damage, EPI, CFS, etc. because there is a double hit by not being able to absorb all the necessary nutrients from the food, and secondly, because more is required in order to heal.

The key with food and water quality intake is to reduce the insults to the body, and increase the nutrients as much as possible. This will help the healing process. Initially it is best to really get strict with your diet and lifestyle, by removing anything that may increase oxidative stress and inflammation. This includes the very obvious smoking and alcohol. But, if you suffer from other elements that can hamper nutrient absorption and healing, such as acid reflux, SIBO and yeast overgrowth, this will need to be tackled as well. These will be covered in the next chapter. Once your microbiome is better balanced, digestion and absorption of food has improved, food sensitivities have lowered and you are in better overall health, you can slowly reintroduce certain foods to see how the body reacts.

Initially there is so much noise, pain, discomfort, and systemic inflammation that it is hard to know which element you should avoid due to a food sensitivity or allergy, versus a temporary issue. Some diet element changes will be for life, depending on how bad the pancreas is damaged. Other actions might only be necessary for a couple of months during the reset phase, or until your lab numbers, as well as your overall feeling of health, are much improved.

When you have been feeling ill for so long, what is two or three months of trying something different, even if it may seem a bit tough initially? Think of a motivator that works for you, whether it is lower pain, lower malaise, ability to do something you have not been to in a while, more energy, etc.

Water Improvement Actions

Let's start with the easy one to fix, and that is the quality of your daily water intake. Tap water quality can be quite unhealthy due to poor infrastructure, bad filtration and all the copiously added toxins. Over time, bad quality water is damaging to the body as it helps destroy the good bacteria in your intestines causing microbiome dysbiosis. It also increases oxidative stress and inflammation due to the toxins the body has to process.

On top of toxins that are not filtered out properly, added chemicals coming out of your tap can include:

• **Fluoride**: A toxic by-product from, for example, the fertilizer industry, often in the form of hydrofluorosilicic acid (HFSA).

• **Chlorine**: A disinfectant that kills bacteria and makes tap water taste and smell like swimming pool water.

• **Chloramines**: A corrosive combination of ammonia and chlorine that is cheaper and more potent than chlorine by itself.

In certain countries where filtration and infrastructure is good, and fluoride, chlorine and chloramines are not added or found coming out of the tap, this health improvement action is obviously not necessary.

<u>So what can you do?</u>

Step 1. The most effective option is to order a bottled water service that delivers to your home, preferably from glass and not plastic bottles. Whilst waiting for the service to start, buy glass bottled mineral water from the store.

Step 2. In restaurants, avoid chlorinated ice and tap water as much as you can. Ask for glass bottled mineral water, or bring your own bottle instead.

Step 3. Avoid plastic contamination as much as you can due to all the plastic particles and leached chemicals that your body has to process, which is another source of oxidative stress. Remember that BPA is only one of the many unhealthy chemicals, so a BPA-free container does not mean free of leached chemicals or small plastic particles.

Step 4. Add a carbon filter in the shower to avoid breathing in the chlorine fumes. A carbon filter is not going to be enough for drinking water, as it will not filter out toxins like added fluoride and other nasties.

Reverse Osmosis

Reverse osmosis (RO) is another often used option, but it is far from optimal as it removes the essential minerals and trace elements we need. It is a wasteful and expensive process, often with plastic components, and requires frequent servicing to remain effective. If you do use RO, or buy water from an RO water shop, please make sure to use a version where essential minerals are added back in. There are at least twenty-one known essential minerals. RO water can also be called demineralized or mineral-poor, which can impact your electrolyte balances and is frankly unhealthy to drink. In the Appendix I have listed a World Health Organization (WHO) report on the dangers of this. Too often I hear the marketing message that we don't get our minerals from water, but through food. Normally we would get up to 5% of certain essential minerals and trace elements from water, some of which are better absorbed if coming from water than from food. Even desalination plants used in some cities stabilize their water with minerals. Now, if you supplement essential minerals, drinking RO water is likely still better for you than unfiltered, chlorinated, fluoridated tap water.

Food Improvement Actions

"Let food be thy medicine…"

Hippocrates

A cliché quote supposedly by the ancient philosopher perhaps, but it is as if you have to become an expert in biochemistry and nutrition to help yourself get better when suffering from pancreas damage and EPI.

Food changes are more difficult to tackle especially when you have no energy to begin with, but also because "diets" are almost impossible to maintain. It is especially tough when there are addictions to, for example, sugar or alcohol, allergies, or sensitivities involved. There is also a tremendous amount of noise surrounding food, with stealth marketing and new health recommendations in the news on a daily basis, making it difficult to determine what to believe. This chapter is based on my trial and error experiences with all the actions that helped me become functional again. Always listen closely to how your body reacts to food and apply common sense regarding your own personal situation.

Let me split food intake into three separate paths depending on your situation:

1. SIBO or Candida Yeast Balancing Food

If you suffer from either small intestinal bacterial overgrowth (SIBO) or yeast overgrowth, refer to Chapter 7 for additional temporary food actions. You can notice quick improvements.

2. Acid or Silent Reflux Balancing Food

This is a symptom which can cause nasty health issues if left untreated, and is often related to food and drink quality as well as SIBO and Candida. Please refer to Chapter 7 for the acid reflux balancing actions if you suffer from it.

3. Pancreas Damage Healing Food

The focus of this chapter is less a diet, but more of a lifestyle that helped me to improve health and healing. Most points are valid for anyone interested in longevity, staving off illness and overall quality of life. The actions listed can impact both the endocrine and exocrine side of the pancreas, as well systemic inflammation, oxidative stress, and the rest of the body. Much of it is obvious, and many elements are from the primal, Okinawan, Mediterranean, or paleo lifestyles. As is always the case, your situation might have specific exceptions due to allergies, sensitivities or other health issues.

In my case I had to tackle all three areas. There are a number of common elements across all three, which makes it a little easier, with the SIBO, Candida and acid reflux balancing actions being a bit stricter, but also temporary.

Pancreas Damage Healing Food Actions

During the initial reset of your diet you will need to be very strict for at least two to three months before slowly re-introducing certain food elements. Some points are beneficial for the rest of your life, but others you can indulge in once in a while, depending on how your body reacts to them. These action items can help reduce overall inflammation, lower the stress on your pancreas, rebuild your microbiome, give your intestines some time to heal and reduce sensitivities in the process. Be tough and honest.

Pay now for the highest quality fresh organic food, or pay later for expensive doctors' visits. But, it does not stop there. Below is a list of over thirty actions I implemented with vital health benefits. They are not necessarily in order of importance.

1. No alcohol. This is for many a tough one, but it is a huge cause of pancreatic damage and oxidative stress. Continue drinking alcohol when you have pancreatic damage and you can make things much worse. My body had given me strong signals years prior that alcohol was to be avoided, so I had not had a drop in many years before my diagnosis. There are some good alcohol free beers available these days that might be worth trying when in better health.

2. No sodas. These contain chemicals, GMO/glyphosate /atrazine herbicide sprayed sugar in excessive levels, and ingredients such as bromated vegetable oils (illegal in the European Union as a food additive), color and flavor chemicals. Diet versions are no better due to the chemicals and fake sugar impact. Also avoid the packaged energy, coffee, post-exercise, sport electrolyte drinks. Some are heavily marketed as "healthy", but are full of harmful chemicals, and excessive levels of artificial and other sugars under various names.

3. Limit sugar. Cut down sugar in all its forms. This will be tough in the beginning and can even cause some temporary withdrawal symptoms. Pretty quickly you will be amazed at how sweet natural things you previously did not find sweet will taste, which is the natural and healthy way. Your system and taste buds will have been desensitized to excess sugar over time. Pay close attention to the ingredients list of the food you buy, and certainly do not add it to your own drinks or food. It is inflammatory, whether it is called agave syrup, honey, dextrose, fructose, corn syrup, fruit juice, lactose, milk powder, cane sugar or juice, ethyl maltol, caramel, glucose, malt, maltodextrin, sorbitol, treacle, molasses, natural sweetener, brown sugar, or maple syrup. Once you are no longer diabetic or pre-diabetic, and have your HbA1c levels around 5.2% or lower, you can of course treat yourself once in a while. But just make yourself aware of all the excessive levels of hidden sugars in restaurant food, packaged food, fast food, canned food and especially most drinks. Also educate yourself on the glycemic index of foods to understand the possible hit to your pancreas a specific food item can have. You don't want high glucose or large insulin spikes in your blood, as it leads to insulin resistance and can do damage to your body over time.

4. No artificial sugar. Avoid any artificial sugars like aspartame, acesulfame potassium, saccharin or sucralose. Many of the artificial sugars have been reported in studies to be linked to microbiome dysbiosis, diabetes, liver damage, obesity, etc. Stevia I do not like due to the lingering taste, but there is conflicting information on its health impact.

5. No candy, bars or sweets. It is sugar under another name. Once my pre-diabetes was resolved and many of the sensitivities subsided, I did bring back, in very limited quantity some organic baked items, gelato and high quality chocolate as an occasional treat. Avoid anything with chemicals, preservatives, high fructose corn syrup, coloring, or anything non-organic. These include the often marketed as "healthy" treats like granola, dried fruit, protein and nut bars, trail mix, frozen yoghurt, etc., which may sound okay until you read the ingredients and see the amounts of sugar.

6. Only organic (Bio or biological in Europe). Do as much as you can to reduce exposure to glyphosate, 2,4D, atrazine and other nasty herbicides and pesticides, as well as excessively used preventative antibiotics and growth hormone, e.g., rBGH or rBST. Even produce and products labelled organic likely still have small amounts of GMO/glyphosate/atrazine herbicides and pesticides due to cross contamination. Officially they can have up to 10% GMO or non-organic and still be labelled as non-GMO or organic. The "non-GMO" label is a bit deceptive, as it does not mean organic and likely still contains nasty herbicides and pesticides. For example, labeling wheat products as non-GMO is sneaky as at the moment wheat is always non-GMO, and is still sprayed with the same herbicides. Also keep in mind that organic does not mean pesticide-free, instead it is a different controlled list of allowed non-synthetic herbicides and pesticides.

7. Dairy. Some dairy is fine if you are not sensitive, but avoid low- or non-fat milk. Not so much for it being dairy, but the sugar (lactose is sugar) content, and often the cows are fed antibiotics, GMO herbicide sprayed corn and soy animal feed. Low fat milk has fewer micronutrients and spikes glucose and insulin more than full fat, thus giving your pancreas an extra hit.

• Organic, grass-fed, antibiotics-free dairy such as plain unsweetened yoghurt or kefir with active bacteria cultures, butter or hard cheeses are good.

• Full-fat buttermilk is fermented, contains lactic acid, vitamins, minerals and beneficial bacteria, and is a lesser known classic that is good for you.

• Careful with milk based protein powder as it is processed, often with chemicals and other ingredients, and it is hard to know the source. Single ingredient organic whey may be an option if you are not sensitive to milk proteins, or choose organic plant based.

• Make sure you are not sensitive to either or both milk proteins; casein or whey. If you are sensitive to a specific milk protein, you can experiment with casein-free, lactose-free or whey-free versions.

• If you are lactose intolerant make sure to add lactase enzyme pills to avoid further irritation, bloating and intestinal distress whenever consuming lactose containing milk products. The level of sensitivity will be personal and is easily determined.

• The easiest way to know if you are sensitive to any elements is to remove dairy completely for a couple of weeks, before slowly introducing one potential irritant at a time. For a while I was sensitive to whey, casein and lactose. Now that my microbiome is more in balance, I only need to take lactase enzymes with some yoghurt, but it was a lot worse for a while. Hard cheese barely has any lactose at all, so you might not need a pill for it.

• Micronutrients that dairy can provide include vitamins A, B1, B2, B6, B9, B12, C, D, E, K, calcium, phosphor, iron, potassium, magnesium, zinc, omega-3 as well as probiotics.

8. Limit packaged, processed and canned goods. During the initial dietary reset avoid these completely and only eat fresh, whole foods. They are often full of GMO/glyphosate/ atrazine ingredients, non-organic, include processed wheat products, chemicals, colorings, preservatives, bulking agents, bad fats and excessive sugar. When things have improved you can add some items back in, but carefully look at all the ingredients on the package. If it contains chemical gibberish, excess sugar in any form, or hydrogenated fats, avoid. Cans have a plastic lining and are usually full of added preservatives, so I would avoid those. Frozen microwave dinners are an obvious no. The only exception I make now is for cans of sardines in water, as they are hard to find otherwise. Avoid most condiments, salad dressings, spreads, and sprays for the same content reasons. Certainly avoid those in plastic containers. Also minimize fresh vegetables that are already prepared and cut, and in plastic containers. I read that some are even washed in sugary water as a preservative. Your body needs to expend energy detoxifying any products you ingest that are not nutrients. Energy is scarce when suffering from EPI.

9. Cereals. Temporarily completely avoid all cereals. Most contain excess sugar content, GMO/glyphosate/atrazine ingredients, preservatives, have any nutrient rich ingredients like the wheat germ removed, and include bleaching, coloring and other chemical processes. They can also contain phytates that can bind with essential minerals like zinc, leading to insufficiencies. Ignore the nefarious marketing messages that make them seem healthy. For a while I thought oatmeal was still a good option until I realized how much it spiked my glucose and insulin, and how much glyphosate is in them. Check out the Environmental Working Group and some of their reports on glyphosate levels in cereals, which is just the tip of the iceberg. Now there are some exceptions becoming available with organic chia, quinoa, buckwheat or hemp alternatives. Just be careful with how it impacts your blood sugar and read the ingredients very carefully. Once your body is in better balance, you could carefully try versions that are organic, whole grain, unbleached, chemicals- and preservative-free, and with no sugar in any form added. Closely pay attention to any inflammation, blood glucose spikes, or bloating signals.

10. Limit restaurants. During the initial dietary reset avoid eating out completely, as many restaurants are diabetes and inflammation factories. When things have improved you can add some back in, but very slowly, infrequently, and be very careful about where they source their ingredients. Check whether they use organic, antibiotics-free ingredients, olive oil, etc. To this day I still have to be extremely careful, and it is rare to find a restaurant which my body can handle. Certainly most chain restaurants are still out of the question for me due to being non-organic. Ingredients often include GMO industrialized seed oils, excessive amounts of sugar, corn and soy fed meat, GMO/glyphosate/atrazine sprayed, highly processed, cheap materials. Be very cautious even with places that market themselves as healthy, vegetarian or vegan-friendly, as they often use the same unhealthy ingredients. Make sure to ask for ceramic or glass for drinks to avoid as much plastic exposure as you can. Avoid chlorinated tap water and ice cubes, and go for a glass bottle of mineral water instead, or bring your own.

11. No fast food. Micronutrient-poor, non-organic, full of chemicals, GMO/glyphosate/atrazine sprayed ingredients, excessive sugar and refined carbs, unhealthy and cheaply sourced fats and protein, and additional toxins through coated paper and plastics exposure. It is a quick dose of oxidative stress.

12. Limit industrialized oils. These include soy, corn, canola (rapeseed), and sunflower oils, which tie directly to one of the reasons to limit restaurant and packaged foods. They are mostly GMO, glyphosate and atrazine sprayed ingredients with chemical and heat processing. They are linked to mitochondrial dysfunction and diabetes to name a few nasties. Stick to organic, extra virgin cold pressed olive oil and, for a bit of variation and in moderation, a little grass-fed butter or ghee (if not sensitive), avocado or coconut oil.

13. Gluten. During the initial dietary reset avoid anything with gluten completely. This includes all wheat types such as einkorn, spelt, semolina, durum, triticale, malt, rye, or barley. You might be surprised to see how ubiquitous wheat products are as cheap filler in everything from sauces (even many soy), condiments, pasta, soups, packaged and canned goods. Once your microbiome is better balanced, and you do not have celiac disease, you can try to reintroduce gluten foods in small amounts to see how your body reacts.

• When your microbiome is imbalanced you are lacking the good bacteria that help break down gluten, so even if you do not have celiac disease, gluten can cause inflammation issues.

• Gluten can be mistaken by the immune system as an invader like Candida yeast or bacteria, causing an immune reaction to gluten. This is another reason to test for microbiome dysbiosis.

• Microbiome dysbiosis and auto-immune reactions are likely a big cause for the increase in gluten sensitivities these days. It is also referred to as non-celiac gluten sensitivity (NCGS).

• Most wheat is non-organic and thus sprayed with glyphosate-based or other synthetic pesticides and herbicides. This is now a worldwide issue.

• There can be many chemicals and bleaching processes used on wheat and wheat products.

• Over 80% of wheat is the endosperm, which is mostly starch and thus considered as glucose to your body. Going gluten-free can temporarily reduce your carbohydrate intake, which helps heal, provided that you do not substitute it with other carbs.

• Be careful with "gluten-free" advertised products as they often contain even more sugar, high glycemic index flour replacements, and other non-organic ingredients to avoid.

14. Bread. Wheat bread is something to cut out completely during the reset diet the first few months. After the reset phase, and if you are feeling better, less inflamed, with a more balanced microbiome, and you do not have celiac disease, you could have another look at bread in limited quantity. A few points to keep in mind about bread:

• Only eat organic, unbleached, whole grain, without added sugar. There are some great artisan type bakeries popping up nowadays, using old-school techniques and just a handful of ingredients, without any preservatives or chemicals.

• Gluten-free bread is not always the answer either since it can be filled with sugar, chemicals and high glycemic replacements for wheat. It also can lack many of the nutrients the wheat germ provides. Make paleo bread at home, or if you buy it, check the ingredients and make sure there is no added sugar in any form.

• The main issues are with the modern types of wheat, the processing, the removal of nutrient-rich wheat germ for shelf life, the bleaching, and before all that the drenching in herbicides. The desiccating of crops refers to spraying the crop with glyphosate based herbicides prior to harvesting, as it ripens faster and is easier to harvest. You cannot wash this off the crops. It is inside the wheat and can impact your microbiome, as well as lower the nutrient and amino acid levels of the wheat.

• Wheat can naturally be high in phytates which bind to minerals, and can reduce the available zinc and other minerals for necessary functions in your body. But, depending on how the baker processes and bakes, these phytates levels can be reduced.

• Mold in grains is not well regulated, so if your system is already struggling, this can be another reason to avoid wheat temporarily.

• Lactobacillus and Bifidobacterium bacteria in your intestines help breakdown phytates and help with gluten digestion. This is another reason why it is important to stop with wheat initially. Reintroduce it only when your microbiome is better balanced so the good intestinal bacteria can help digest it.

• Reintroduce wheat only in small amounts to see how your body reacts and pay close attention to any signals your body is giving you, such as inflammation, tiredness, mind fog, bloating, itching, fingertip or face swelling, joint pain or swelling.

• The bran and germ contain most of the valuables, and if prepared properly, bread can contain essential amino acids, choline, omega fatty acids, fiber, phytonutrients, vitamins A, B1, B2, B3, B5, B6, B8, B9, B11, B12, C, D, E, K, and minerals like calcium, iron, iodine, potassium, phosphorous, copper, magnesium, zinc, and selenium. Depending on the type of salt (e.g., European baker's), minerals such as iodine can be added. Often nuts and seeds are added to the bread as well, adding omega fatty acids.

• Wheat is usually a good source of tryptophan, but it has to be organic to avoid the glyphosate herbicide impact on amino acids like tryptophan.

• If bread is not old and hard within two days of buying it, do not buy it again. It means that it was not made in a healthy manner, with the whole grain that includes the nutrients, and without cheap preservatives like sugar. I slice and freeze most of the loaf as soon as I buy it, as it keeps longer. It only takes a few minutes to defrost and still tastes quite fresh.

The paleo community generally frowns upon grains and bread, but I think the underlying reasons for potential harm need to be looked at more closely. These include, the generally high added sugar content, the non-organic glyphosate impact on the wheat itself and our microbiome, the removal of the nutrient dense wheat germ and the fiber rich bran or husk, the chemical and bleaching treatments, the baker's preparation methods, the added preservatives, the microbiome issues of the general population and subsequent issues with breaking down gluten and phytates. Also the sheer volume consumed, often unwittingly through its usage as cheap filler in many packaged goods, is an issue.

Organic, whole grain wheat bread can be an amazing potential source of nutrients if you understand the possible microbiome dysbiosis link, underlying issues and caveats. I sometimes take a probiotic a few minutes before my meal to boost bacteria to help break down gluten. Just like I will have a lactase pill before having yoghurt, a probiotic seems to help with bread. But, even though my microbiome is able to handle bread again, it is still a moderation type of food, and at maximum I might have a few slices every other day.

15. Pasta. Often made with non-organic, processed wheat flour, devoid of most of the nutrients and fiber for extended shelf life. This is one of the easiest things to replace with alternative ingredient versions like quinoa, buckwheat or lentils where you will not miss the wheat. Just make sure it is organic, and not filled with other chemicals or high-glycemic index wheat replacements.

16. Vegan and vegetarian. If you are vegan or vegetarian be careful with getting all the essential micronutrients that you can miss out on, or not get in sufficient quantities to heal. Be sure to monitor your levels and supplement when necessary, essentials such as calcium, iron, zinc, omega-3 fatty acids, iodine, choline, selenium, vitamins B2, B12 and D3. And of course, stick with only organic. A benefit of being vegan or vegetarian is that you are already very aware of the dangers of the food supply, but be careful with all the fake meat products. Packaged vegan products are often touted as healthy, but when you read the ingredients they can be full of sugar, industrial GMO oils, chemicals and non-organic, herbicide sprayed fillers.

17. Soup. Eat only homemade, never canned. I ate chicken, vegetable, and bone broth soup for lunch every day for years. Bone broth is very healing. For months this was all I could even tolerate. Prep a week's worth of soup using a slow-pressure cooker, and add lots of various fresh vegetables on top at serving time. Here is a simple recipe that I still eat almost daily:

• Base: organic grass-fed beef or air chilled organic chicken, carrots, celery, onion, spring onion, zucchini, garlic, one potato, limited wild rice, variety of mushrooms, organic bone broth, variety of salts (Hawaiian red, Himalayan pink, A. Vogel herb salt), herbs such as bay leaf, basil, thyme, rosemary, and parsley to taste.

• Before eating and during the slow reheating, I will add a few extra vegetables such as Swiss chard, beet, endive, watercress, kale, jicama, bakchoi, broccoli, cauliflower, asparagus, arugula, fennel, or micro greens. Do not boil. Sometimes I add a little bit of olive oil after serving.

• Often I have half an avocado on the side with some curry powder, pepper (careful with your sensitivities) and Himalayan pink salt.

• Change ingredients and spices to your sensitivities and taste preferences, just make sure to use high quality ingredients.

18. Salt. Only use high quality mineral rich salt such as Himalayan pink, Celtic sea or A. Vogel Herbamare salt. By avoiding restaurant and packaged foods, which contain a surprising amount of low-quality, high-sodium, bleached, and de-mineralized salt, you need to make sure you consume enough good quality salt in your cooking. Or even have a plain pinch if you crave it. High sodium pushes out magnesium and potassium. This is another reason to avoid demineralized table salt, which is bleached, with sugar and chemicals added, is and mostly sodium chloride. Those with RO water setups will likely also require more, as they miss out on essential minerals and trace elements.

19. Herbs. There are many herbs to use in cooking or in tea, which provide phytonutrients and help in healing. The important thing is to slowly introduce them, as in the beginning you might be sensitive to many like I was. Once your microbiome has balanced a bit and you have resolved some of the big items, you might notice improvements in sensitivities. However, I still have to watch out with paprika, pepper, chili and peppermint for example, so listen to your body's reaction. Below are a few notable ones to consider:

- Oregano, curcumin, coriander, saffron, turmeric, ginger, fennel, black pepper, cinnamon, coriander, cloves, ginger, garlic, cinnamon, basil, peppermint, echinacea, chamomile, aloe vera, sage, nettle, lemon grass, nutmeg, and chili.

20. Vegetables, healthy carbs. Buy fresh, unprepared, uncut, and as many, as colorful, and as big a variety as you can handle. It is the best source of antioxidants, healthy calories, amino acids, phytonutrients, vitamins, and minerals. Be careful with, and eat in moderation any high starch and high glycemic index vegetables like rice and potatoes, as these are seen as sugar to the body. They can spike glucose and insulin levels. I unscientifically use the palm of my hand as a guideline to determine the maximum amount of potato or wild rice for the day, and many days will go without.

21. Legumes. A group of vegetables which include peanuts, beans, and peas are generally frowned upon by the paleo community. The antinutrients phytic acid (called phytate when bound to a mineral) and lectins (damage intestinal lining and can cause an autoimmune reaction) are found in legumes. Some also have a high glycemic index. Very careful preparation is needed, which includes soaking twelve plus hours and cooking them properly. This removes most of these antinutrients. Legumes are prebiotic, have many essential vitamins and minerals. Fermented beans like natto are healthy, but personally am not a fan. Take your microbiome balance into consideration, as good gut bacteria can help break down phytates. If you are out of balance, you will have a harder time digesting legumes. Perhaps wait until you are a bit stronger to reintroduce legumes, and try using a probiotic before the meal to help with the breakdown. I still have to be careful with this category, including peanuts. Listen to your body.

22. Healthy fats. This includes items like seeds, nuts, avocado, olives, eggs, small fish, grass-fed dairy and meat. There are some sites and books that still mention a low-fat diet, but that has been debunked and can slow down your healing. Often the classic advice you read is to go low-fat when you have pancreas issues. Why would you remove a crucial healing element (essential fatty acids) from your diet, but continue to eat processed grains, low-fat dairy, and sugar laden juices that continue inflaming your body? You need to alleviate the burden on the pancreas, but through pancreatic enzyme replacement therapy so that you can break down the food, including the essential fats. Limit bad fats like trans, hydrogenated and GMO "vegetable" oils. Limit grain-, soy- and corn-fed meat and dairy fat, and only eat organically sourced. Quality is important, as toxins are stored in fat not just in our bodies, but also in the fat of the animals we eat.

23. Healthy protein. For the complete amino acids requirement, proteins from vegetables, seeds and nuts are great. Seeds like chia are rich in tryptophan, and rice and beans combined provide most of the essential amino acids. For many other micronutrients, animal protein is also important, just know the source of your protein. Buy organic and pasture-raised whenever possible. Eggs should be from happy, organic, pasture raised chickens that were not fed soy or corn. Avoid unhappy, cage raised, GMO, glyphosate, atrazine and antibiotics fed, chlorine-washed chickens. Free-range is a marketing slogan and is not much better than cage raised. Beef should come from grass-fed and grass-finished, organic, antibiotics- and hormone-free cows. Avoid non-organic farmed fish, as they are fed GMO grains and antibiotics. Limit processed meat due to non-organic ingredients, fillers, chemicals and added sugar preservatives.

Don't eat too much protein, as your body can transform it into glucose through gluconeogenesis. This is how your body turns protein into glycogen that can be used as glucose to burn for fuel when needed. The WHO mentions 0.83 grams of protein per day for each kilogram of body weight to keep the lights on, assuming a perfect amino acid balance. One gram per kilogram of body weight is what I roughly use as a guideline per day. But, temporarily we might need more to heal, and those with EPI will not absorb everything optimally and might need a little more.

24. Choline. Check your choline intake since it has a large effect on your methylation cycle, homocysteine levels, neurotransmitters through acetylcholine, and accumulation of fat and cholesterol in the liver. Those with EPI are likely deficient in lecithin, choline and subsequently metabolites like betaine and phosphatidylcholine. Add some choline rich foods like wheat germ, eggs, grass-fed dairy, and beef liver or shrimp to your diet.

25. Primal or Paleo. There are many great elements to implement from this anti-inflammatory and healing lifestyle. It helped me heal, lower systemic inflammation, resolve pre-diabetes and hypoglycemic episodes. In the Appendix I have listed some great information on the subject.

• Read up on primal and paleo diets, and no, paleo does not mean just eat lots of meat! Check out Mark Sisson and his wealth of information in books, podcasts and websites.

• It recommends a balanced lifestyle, avoiding excess, enjoying full-body exercise, enjoying the outdoors and sunshine, eating lots of nutrient dense vegetables of a great variety, healthy proteins, healthy oils, moderation of starches and carbs, limited full fat dairy, no grains and healthy fats.

• Reduce you sugar, starch and processed carbohydrate consumption and dependency. 100-150 grams of carbohydrates per day are considered a healthy level by the primal community, but can vary depending on your goal and exercise levels.

• Become fat adapted and change from being a "sugar burner". This means that your body uses its own fat storage easily as an efficient fuel, and you are no longer addicted to sugar and carbs.

• Paleo does warn about a few food groups such as legumes, dairy and grains. However, the core reasons for being careful with these food groups needs to be considered, as they can provide a lot of essential nutrients. Some points to consider are the sheer volume of grains generally consumed, where they are sourced and grown, the non-organic glyphosate and atrazine effects, how they are prepared, and importantly the state of your microbiome. Having enough beneficial bacteria to help break down elements like lactose, gluten, and phytates is crucial.

26. Ketogenic Diet. A very popular anti-inflammatory diet at the moment. But those with EPI need to be very cautious, as you likely are already nutrient deficient. The liver either produces cholesterol, which is used to store energy amongst many other things, or ketones endogenously from your adipose fat if in a fasted state. Insulin and glucagon hormones produced in the pancreas will stop ketone production so that the body uses up glucose. But, if you are following the points listed in this chapter, or follow a paleo or primal lifestyle, you already produce ketones. A 12-14 hour fast per day, which should be standard anyway, can help get you into nutritional ketosis. Ketones have potent healing qualities and are linked to helping with mitochondrial dysfunction. I have used a device from KetoMojo which checks ketones in the blood. Urine strips or breath test versions are not as accurate. My ketone blood level was between 0.4 and 1.7 (mmol/L) before breakfast, just by following my regular diet, and eating within a 10-12 hour window.

Some people seem to take this diet to the extreme, and in addition add exogenous (i.e., not made in the body) ketone salts through supplements. Ketoacidosis, just one of the possible side effects, is life threatening. I also avoid the exogenous ketone supplements at this time as they are often hyped up, filled with flavoring, coloring and preservative chemicals, as well as excess sugars often hidden in innocent sounding labels. The ones I tried spiked my blood sugar level considerably and made me feel ill.

27. Timing. How and when you eat has an impact on your pancreas and your body.

• Avoid constant snacking, as each time you give your pancreas a hit by getting it to try to produce enzymes and insulin. It needs rest in order to heal.

• Eat in a 10-12 hour window each day, and stay consistent with the timing of your meals and snacks.

• More stringent fasting and intermittent fasting needs to be considered very carefully, since those with EPI are already so low on nutrients and calories. Intermittent fasting is normally very healthy. It gives the pancreas amongst other things a rest and time to heal. It helps your body clean up dead and sick cells, and it promotes ketone production in the liver. Once you are much stronger this could be looked at, but initially I would stick with the 10-12 hour eating window.

• Mindful eating. This is not some philosophical advice, although mindful eating is healthy. But, you do produce some enzymes through saliva to breakdown carbs, and chewing longer mixes it better. The smaller the bits are that your stomach acid and pancreatic enzymes need to break down, the more nutrients you will be able to get from them.

• The order in which you eat carbs matters in the insulin spike. It is better to eat some protein or fat first and wait a few minutes before carbs like starch or rice. Your body releases an enzyme which slows down the stomach processes for protein or fat. This way carbs are released more slowly into the system causing less high insulin spikes.

• There was the eat-many-small-meals-per-day fad, which is not helpful. Give your intestines and pancreas a rest.

• Try to walk after a meal, as it helps reduce glucose in the blood by using it in muscles, instead of needing the pancreas to work harder on an insulin spike.

28. Exclusion diets. Be careful with any fad exclusionary diets. I noticed the impact of nutrient deficiencies with nutritional tests by excluding, e.g., legumes, dairy or wheat, or by going gluten-free for too long. Temporarily, during the dietary reset, or when healing from systemic inflammation, SIBO or Candida, you have to be strict before re-introducing elements. There are valid reasons for, and visible physical impacts from some temporary exclusion diets, but sometimes the root cause for a symptom is not completely understood. Or people go to extremes. Many of these fads start in the United States, but are really a reaction to the symptoms of the quality of the standard, highly processed diet with its tremendous amounts of sugar, bad fat and oil, GMO glyphosate and atrazine sprayed products, fluoridated and chlorinated tap water, and all the impacts on our microbiome.

29. Limit plastic exposure. Plastic exposure is impossible to avoid completely these days, as it is used on almost all packaging products. It is found in tap and plastic bottled water, and even in fish. Try hard to do as much as you can, as you can ingest plastic particles and leached chemicals like phthalates, BPA, BPF, BPS, PFC, or PVC. Even "healthy" producers and grocery stores that you trust surprisingly use a lot of toxic packaging. These are more toxic, oxidative stress, hits to the body you do not need!

30. Fruit. Really limit your fruit intake. A few berries, half a banana, avocado or apple per day would be my maximum. It is an inefficient way to get enough vitamin C, especially during the healing period, when you need a high dosage of antioxidants. The sugar level is simply too high in most fruit, so it affects your glucose and insulin levels.

31. Avoid juices. Even if freshly squeezed, just look at how many oranges or apples you need to squeeze for just one glass. And even worse, avoid completely any store or restaurant bought fruit or vegetable juices, fruit shakes, or smoothies. Just look at the mostly non-organic ingredients with shocking amounts of sugar (similar amounts as soft drinks), added chemicals and preservatives, and surprising countries of origin. They are unhealthy, inflammatory, and insulin spiking. Ignore the loud and dishonest marketing messages. Have a little bit of whole fruit or some berries instead, which will be a smaller dose of sugar and include healthy fiber. Even smoothies should only be home-made and without juices and sugars, and a very limited amount of real whole fruit.

32. Grains and starches. It is tied to a few of the elements and reasons to limit these that were already discussed above, such as bread, cereals, gluten, pasta, healthy carbs and proteins. Limit your grains and starches more strictly during the initial reset of your diet, and until you see improvement in glucose and insulin lab results. Your body views these as glucose for energy production or energy storage. Some starches have a high glycemic index and will spike your insulin considerably, such as instant oatmeal, cereals, white rice, corn, white bread, and many potato types. You can look at replacing those with lower glycemic index versions. But, work on becoming a "fat-burner" instead of "sugar-burner" first. This is when you are not so dependent on glucose/sugar/refined carbs, and your body is efficient at utilizing its own fat storage for fuel. The primal lifestyle links in the appendix have good information on this. Now that my intestinal system and microbiome is more balanced, I eat small amounts in moderation. But I stick with limited whole grain and organic versions. I also still check the blood glucose meter occasionally to see the impact and check or estimate my HbA1c level.

33. Drink. Stick with clean, filtered, non-chlorinated, non-fluoridated water, tea, and coffee, and if you can handle it, a little full-fat buttermilk for the beneficial intestinal bacteria. Especially during the healing period, stay strict with drinks and avoid anything with sugar or chemicals in it, or from plastic containers.

34. A.G.E. Foods. Reduce foods containing really high levels of advanced glycation end-products (AGE) during the healing period, as they cause oxidative stress. Once you feel better you can reintroduce some high AGE items just because they taste so good and might make you feel happier, but of course in moderation. Bacon is very high in AGE, but tastes so good I will treat myself once in a while. Again, know how it was sourced and processed, avoid those with added sugars and chemicals, organic only, and know what the animals were fed. Be careful not to get oil to a smoking point when cooking, as this also introduces unnecessary AGEs.

35. Read labels carefully. Just because something is labelled organic, gluten-free, natural (a completely meaningless label), non-GMO, natural flavoring (not natural), low-fat, diet, reduced-sugar, it does not mean it actually contains healthy amounts of sugar or is good for you. Non-GMO does not mean organic. Read the labels carefully and you might be shocked at the sheer amount of ingredients listed, such as chemicals, meaningless jargon included to hide those chemicals, fillers, coloring, flavoring and preservatives. Also be aware of the packaging materials used, for example, the type of plastic or coated paper, as toxins can leach into your food and drinks as well. Do your homework, but this is why, during the reset portion of your diet and the healing period, it is best to avoid anything packaged or processed.

Summary

Something that helped me, especially in the beginning phase when I was sensitive to almost everything, was to keep a food, beverage and supplement impact journal. This way I could keep track of how my body reacted to all the various tweaks, either positively or negatively, and allow me to go back to see the physical and mental impacts over time.

I have tried to remember all the elements that helped me during my healing process and listed them above, but some might be different for you due to your personal situation, other medical issues, sensitivities or allergies.

Be honest with yourself and keep your common sense. I find it interesting that most of the food related points above would be considered a no-brainer, and just plain common sense by our parents and grandparents.

Seriously, strictly and honestly address your food and water quality intake, both in terms of reducing bodily insults, as well as providing the necessary nutrients. Your body will thank you, as it can drastically impact your healing process and timeline.

CHAPTER SEVEN

SIBO, Candida, and Reflux

Small intestinal bacterial overgrowth (SIBO), yeast overgrowth like Candida, and acid or silent reflux are linked in their underlying causes, overlapping symptoms, and the possible rebalancing steps.

Those with pancreas damage will likely suffer from one, or all of these, and they need to be addressed to help the body heal.

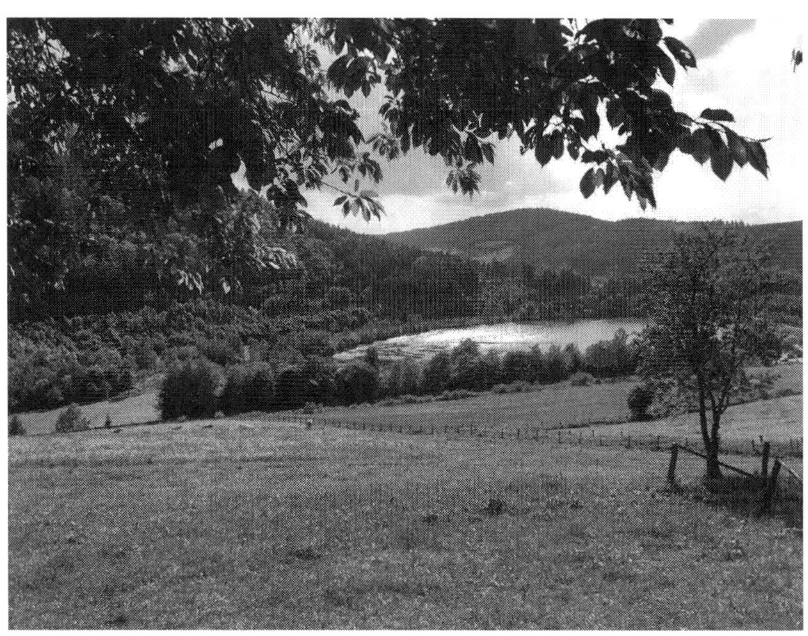

Pancreas damage and EPI often go hand-in-hand with small intestinal bacterial overgrowth (SIBO) and yeast (e.g., Candida) overgrowth issues. An unhealthy diet, with excess sugar and improper digestion of food particles, will allow yeast and bacteria to flourish in areas where they normally would not. This can cause excess toxic byproducts from these dysbiotic bacteria and yeast. These symptoms need to be treated immediately, as it creates a vicious cycle of nutrient deficiencies, not to mention many very unpleasant symptoms. SIBO and yeast overgrowth can create a coating or biofilm in areas that should be relatively clean of bacteria and yeast, such as your esophagus, stomach and duodenum. This can cause nutrient deficiencies, as the biofilm blocks intestinal villi from absorbing nutrients properly, but also because bacteria feeds on the nutrients that your body needs. Keep in mind that you will never get rid of them completely, and that is not the goal, as they are part of a normal microbiome.

Bringing a better balance to the microbiome is the goal, as we need the symbiotic relation with beneficial intestinal bacteria, yeast and fungus.

Common culprits in causing dysbiosis can be:

• Excessive sugar content in food and drinks. Even those thought of as healthy, like fruit and vegetable juices, protein bars, most cereals, granola bars, energy drinks, etc. are important causes.

• Chlorine and chloramines in tap water.

• Glyphosate, an antibiotic and most widely used herbicide, present in non-organic and many packaged food and drinks.

• Antibiotics treatments.

• Insufficient prebiotics and probiotics food elements.

The symptoms are numerous as I outlined in a prior chapter, and resolving these issues can provide a big relief. Functional or integrative medicine doctors often have more experience with resolving this, whereas many standard doctors, including gastroenterologists, often do not take this seriously enough. It is also important to note that it requires a combination of prescription medicine, supplements and diet changes to resolve. Work with your doctor on prescriptions and a specific schedule. Because you are often so weak with pancreas damage effects, it might be better to stagger the treatments of antibiotics and antifungals, but the supplements can be helpful for both. Below are useful actions for both SIBO and Candida, as there is some overlap, but some rebalancing actions are very specific for each ailment.

Diet: Rebalance SIBO and Candida

It is a good idea to, at least temporarily, limit your diet in ways which lowers inflammation and lowers the food desired by yeast and bacteria. If you have ever baked your own bread, you know what a little bit of sugar does with yeast activation and its explosive growth. Please remember, bacteria and yeast love sugar and simple carbohydrates.

This diet is good to implement for the first one to two months in order to set a baseline. It follows the lines of the prior chapter on pancreas healing food, with a few extra temporary restrictions. It includes lots of healthy multi-colored vegetables, healthy proteins, low sugars, limited carbohydrates, healthy dairy, and minimally packaged and processed foods.

Some guidelines are:

- No added sugar in any form, including those often thought of as healthy, like honey. Although Manuka honey does have antimicrobial qualities, I would be careful with it too due to the high sugar content.

- Eat only organic to avoid further hits to the microbiome from, for example, glyphosate herbicides, with its antibiotic function.

• Avoid restaurant and café food to avoid excessive amounts of sugar, industrialized seed oils, cheap non-organic ingredients, and chemicals, all of which you have no control over.

• Gluten-free. This is tough as you will realize how much non-organic wheat is used in many packaged products. It is even in ones you would not expect it, like soy sauce or other condiments. Avoid wheat, barley, spelt, oats, triticale and rye. Gluten-free replacements can include amaranth, buckwheat, quinoa, millet, rice, or sorghum.

• Legumes are fine if they are fresh, not canned, and prepared properly (e.g., long soaking periods to lower antinutrients).

• Avoid milk due to the high sugar (lactose) content. Unsweetened, plain yoghurt which contains healthy live bacteria, cheese, and buttermilk are good to help rebalance.

• Avoid fruit juices, smoothies and vegetable juices due to the high sugar content.

• Avoid sodas of any kind, including sugar-free versions.

• Avoid chlorinated tap water and ice cubes, as you do not want to kill good bacteria.

• Limit fruit. At most eat just one small fresh (not canned, not frozen, not dried) serving of whole fruit per day, preferably berries, avocado or an apple. Avoid citrus, melons, or peaches due to potential mold content and high sugar.

• Avoid alcohol as this is pure sugary fuel for the fire. This should be avoided or limited by anyone with pancreatic damage anyway due to the oxidative stress. Stick with water, herbal teas, and temporarily for Candida treatment only limited coffees (mold content can be an issue here as well).

• Avoid deli meats, canned food, most condiments and just generally limit packaged food.

• Add in some food items which are naturally antibacterial or antifungal, such as coconut oil, cinnamon, curcumin, garlic, clove, oregano, mustard, and thyme.

• Add in food with prebiotic qualities. This is non-digestible fiber that is food for the good bacteria and best taken in through food. For example, garlic, artichoke, leek, onions, jicama root, asparagus, or green banana. With fermented products like sauerkraut, kimchee, natto, atjar, miso, tempeh, chutney, just temporarily avoid any with yeast content or yeast fermented products if going through a Candida rebalancing.

• Avoid anything containing yeast, such as packaged, baked goods, vinegar, pickled items, and condiments. You might be surprised how much is used in packaged goods. This is more relevant for lowering Candida yeast than SIBO.

• Avoid mushrooms (fungus), peanuts (high mold content, aflatoxin), blue cheese (fungus), Marmite (yeast) and dry roasted nuts (sugar). This is more relevant for lowering Candida yeast than SIBO.

Supplements: Rebalance SIBO and Candida

The following supplements can help to rebalance in a multi-pronged approach. Some of the supplements can help reduce the yeast or bacteria. Others can help disrupt the biofilm or the cell wall that protects the bacteria and yeast, so that the antifungal and antibacterial can be more effective. Biofilm is crucial to tackle but very difficult to confirm, even with biopsies. When you see a patch of bacterial growth in nature it is often in a dark film. Picture it as something similar to what happens inside your stomach and intestines. Bacteria manage to hide from your immune system in the biofilm. It can exacerbate deficiencies as the bacteria absorb minerals and vitamins for their food. Other supplements add beneficial bacteria and yeast. Although there is still much unknown at this point on the effectiveness of taking the pills that are not specifically created for your microbiome, the idea behind taking probiotics is to help grow the healthy bacteria back in the emptier "real estate". Supplements to consider are:

Type	Note
Biocidin Advanced Formula by Bio-Botanical Research	Used during the treatment of Candida (4 weeks) and SIBO (3 weeks) as it is a strong botanical agent with many ingredients. 5 drops, 3 times per day with meals and with a slow build up.
Interfase Plus Enzymes by Klaire Labs	Used during the treatment of Candida (4 weeks) and SIBO (3 weeks). This helps disrupt the biofilm of the bacteria and yeast. 2 pills, 3 times per day with meals.
MCT oil from organic coconut	Used daily during the treatment of Candida (4 weeks) and SIBO (3 weeks). The caprylic acid in coconut oil is effective by penetrating the cell walls of yeast, causing it to rupture.
Molybdenum Chelated by Thorne Research	It is used in the body to break down a Candida by-product acetaldehyde, a neurotoxin, which can cause pain and weakness in tissues. Taken daily for 3 months. For Candida treatment only.
Oregano SAP	Sporadic, with food. It is a natural antifungal and an ingredient in Biocidin.
Probio Max DF, Probiotic Complete by Xymogen, Ther-Biotic Complete by Klaire Labs	Probiotics. Used multiple times per day 30 minute prior to a meal during SIBO and Candida rebalancing. Also used daily whenever on an antibiotic treatment. Use a minimum of 10-15 billion count pills to help rebuild good bacteria levels. Take 1-2 hours away from the antibiotics if you are on a course.

Type	Note
Serralase by Klaire Labs	Proteolytic enzymes blend which helps break down food, cellular debris, and supports tissue repair. Daily during the SIBO and Candida treatments. Contains bromelain, papain, catalase, and peptidase enzymes.
Saccharomycin DF by Xymogen	Probiotic yeast (Saccharomyces boulardii). Used almost daily during the treatment of Candida (4 weeks) for microbiome rebalancing. For Candida treatment only.

SIBO Actions

SIBO can cause many symptoms including diarrhea, nausea, acid reflux, burning stomach, gastritis, stomach and intestinal issues, pains, malabsorption, bloating, microbiome dysbiosis, vitamin and mineral deficiencies, skin irritations, leaky gut, hypoglycemia, fatigue, brain fog, blurry eyesight, depression, food and smell sensitivities, headaches, itching, etc. It is worth testing for even though tests are not very accurate. If you have not been breaking down food properly due to a lack of pancreatic enzymes, it is very likely that the bacteria in your system will be out of balance and have flourished in places where they should not have. Follow these four steps to help improve your bacterial balance.

Step 1. SIBO Testing

This is the breath test I took to check for both methane and hydrogen producing bacteria. There are other variations of tests, just be sure to take one that checks for both methane and hydrogen levels.

- **Commonwealth Diagnostics International small intestinal bacterial overgrowth (SIBO)**.

The nutritional organic acid and comprehensive stool tests mentioned in a prior chapter have a dedicated section for bacterial overgrowth indicators. They also indicate potential pathogenic or commensal flora levels and types. The tests will cover both yeast and SIBO.

- **Genova Diagnostics NutrEval FMV** or the **Great Plains Laboratory Nutritional and Metabolic Profile** are both good options to consider.

- **Doctor's Data Comprehensive Stool Analysis**.

Step 2. Antibiotics Treatment

These are two different antibiotics to be used together in a ten day course. Please note that research mentioned that Rifaximin alone is not effective for methane related SIBO. They work more effectively when used together. There are different methane and hydrogen producing bacteria that are impacted differently by the two types of antibiotics. They require a doctor's prescription.

- **Neomycin**

- **Rifaximin** (a.k.a. Xifaxan)

Step 3. SIBO and Candida Rebalancing Diet

Follow the section earlier in the chapter for a strict but temporary diet in order to help your system heal and rebalance. Stop feeding the undesired bacterial colonies.

Step 4. SIBO and Candida Rebalancing Supplements

Follow the section earlier in the chapter for a list of supplements that can help your system heal and rebalance.

Candida Yeast Overgrowth Actions

It is also worth testing for, but if you have not been breaking down food properly due to lack of pancreatic enzymes it is very likely that the fungi (yeast is a type of fungus) in your system will be out of balance, and have flourished in places where they should not have. Candida is well known as dysbiotic yeast, however, it is just one of many fungi that are a natural part of our microbiome. The actions listed will impact not just Candida, but other fungi overgrowths as well. Similar to SIBO, this is another area which I wish I had known about a lot earlier. It can impede healing, can also cause malabsorption, and a whole host of symptoms similar to SIBO. Symptoms can include brain fog, fatigue, urinary tract infections, mood swings, irritability, sugar cravings, depression, bloating, stomach, intestinal and stool issues, smell sensitivity, skin issues, bad breath, muscle and joint pains, itching, mood swings, blurry eyesight, nasal congestion, sugar cravings and acid reflux.

Candida ferments sugars into acetaldehyde, ethanol, ammonia and a few other toxins which your body works very hard to process. I read that a protein found in Candida is very similar to gluten, which can cause your immune system to react to gluten as if it is an invader like Candida. This is another possible connection to the increase in gluten sensitivities found these days, and another reason to resolve a Candida overgrowth issue.

Follow these four steps to help improve your yeast balance.

Step 1. Candida Yeast Testing

The nutritional organic acid and comprehensive stool tests mentioned before have a dedicated section for yeast overgrowth indicators. They also indicate potential pathogenic or commensal flora levels and types. The tests will cover both yeast and SIBO.

• **Genova Diagnostics NutrEval FMV** or the **Great Plains Laboratory Nutritional and Metabolic Profile** are both good options to consider.

- **Doctor's Data Comprehensive Stool Analysis.**

Step 2. Antifungal Treatment

- **Nystatin**

A one month course of one million units per day, from a compounding pharmacy, can help lower the yeast levels. It requires a doctor's prescription. There are also other well-known antifungals like fluconazole, but due to the possible side effects, my doctor did not use those.

Step 3. SIBO and Candida Rebalancing Diet

Follow the section earlier in the chapter for a strict but temporary diet in order to help your system heal and rebalance. Stop feeding the undesired fungal colonies.

Step 4. SIBO and Candida Rebalancing Supplements

Follow the section earlier in the chapter for a list of supplements that can help your system heal and rebalance.

Silent or Acid Reflux Actions

Whether it is the overt pain after eating or drinking version, or the silent reflux version, this is a symptom that should be resolved by diet and not constant symptom suppressing drugs like acid reducers and proton pump inhibitors.

Acid reflux is your body telling you something is likely quite wrong with your food and beverage intake, as well signaling dysbiosis in your stomach and intestines. Of course there might be other medical issues at play that can cause acid or silent reflux, including mechanical ones, so discuss it with your doctor. For example, other related issues I had run into in the past included hiatal hernia or H. Pylori bacteria issues.

Stomach acid goes up through your lower esophageal sphincter muscle into your esophagus, throat and sometimes lungs when this should not normally happen. If you ignore this too long you can get all kinds of serious health issues and complications, including cancer! The action items to consider are:

Step 1. Raise your bed.

The single easiest and very effective thing I did was to elevate the head of my bed by 20-25 cm, which stopped the flow of acid up into my throat at night. Keep the overall bed flat though, so put blocks of wood or a stack of books underneath just the two bed posts at the head of the bed.

Step 2. SIBO and Candida rebalancing.

Follow the earlier sections to test for and tackle SIBO and Candida overgrowth issues, if present. If you have ever seen how sugar interacts with yeast, you understand how bubbles forming in your stomach can cause stomach acid to come up. There is a good chance you have an overgrowth issue if you have acid or silent reflux.

Step 3. Top-down acid reduction.

Temporarily consider a low acid diet for a month. There are many books on the subject, one of which is listed in the Appendix, but below are some easy diet tips. You need to give your esophagus time to calm down. The key is that a digestive enzyme called pepsin comes up into your esophagus during reflux, and it thrives and reactivates on anything acidic. It is supposed to stay in your stomach to help digest your food, not digest your esophagus or throat!

Acid reflux diet tips

- Follow the SIBO and Candida rebalancing diet outlined earlier, as this will help lower key aggravators such as sugar.

• Drink alkaline, non-chlorinated, non-fluoridated water (pH >7).

• Cut down your portion size, at least temporarily, so your stomach does not get overly full.

• Eat all your daily food in a 10-12 hour window, with no late-night eating, drinking (except water), or snacking.

• If you do get some packaged products, check for and avoid those with preservatives like citric acid, phosphoric acid, ascorbic acid or vitamin C.

Cut down on all of the following items, at least during the reflux healing time, in order to give your esophagus, throat and stomach a rest. Once you feel better you can slowly reintroduce those that are not unhealthy. But, watch for any negative symptoms and how your body reacts to them.

• Alcohol
• Caffeine
• Chocolate
• Carbonated, citrus, caffeinated, or sugary drinks
• Canned foods
• Onions
• Raw tomatoes
• Peppermint
• Garlic
• Citrus fruit
• Strawberries
• Sugar and other high-carb food
• Spicy food
• Deep fried food
• Chlorinated tap water and ice cubes
• Processed fatty meats

Step 4. Bottom-up acid reduction.

In conjunction with the first three steps, I took Zantac75 (Ranitidine antacid) three times per day, away from meals and before bed, for three weeks in order to temporarily lower the acid in my stomach and ease the gastritis. I also took the occasional Tums antacid. In addition, some supplements like GI Encap, Glutagenics and L-glutamine helped heal the intestinal lining and lower irritation.

The lowering of acid from both food and beverage intake, as well as from up-flow from the stomach, allowed the pepsins to calm down and actual healing to occur in the stomach, throat and esophagus.

Antacids and PPI

A side note on antacids and proton pump inhibitors (PPI). They should be used cautiously and only for a short period of time due to the potential damage they can do. They certainly should not be used as a way to mask your symptoms, as happens way too much these days. Your stomach acid is crucial. Ironically, many people suffering from acid reflux likely have low stomach acid (i.e., pH levels too high). This can cause improper break down of food, indigestion, malabsorption leading subsequently to nutrient deficiencies, overgrowth of yeast and bacteria. If you do not have the right stomach pH level, your lower esophageal sphincter will not close properly, allowing the stomach contents back up into the esophagus. By taking antacid or PPI pills for long periods of time you are not only not resolving the root cause, but you are making it worse by feeding the yeast and bacteria; a vicious cycle. You are damaging your body from the side effects of those same pills, one of which is low stomach acid (a.k.a. hypochlorhydria).

A simple unscientific test to approximate acid level is by drinking a quarter teaspoon of baking soda (sodium bicarbonate) mixed in a glass of water on an empty stomach in the morning. This creates bubbles within two to three minutes when mixed with the hydrochloric acid in your stomach. If after five minutes nothing happens, there is a very good chance the pH of your stomach acid is too high (i.e., low stomach acid).

CHAPTER EIGHT

Road to Recovery Actions

Practical steps I took to go from death's door to a functioning human being again. This includes areas of focus such as pancreatic enzyme replacement, food and water quality, nutrition deficiencies, SIBO, Candida, reflux, inflammation, oxidative stress, bodily insults, and primal living healing actions.

Anything that helped me in the healing process is covered. Some issues you might not have considered as hampering your healing process, and some actions you might not have considered before as helpful to your overall health.

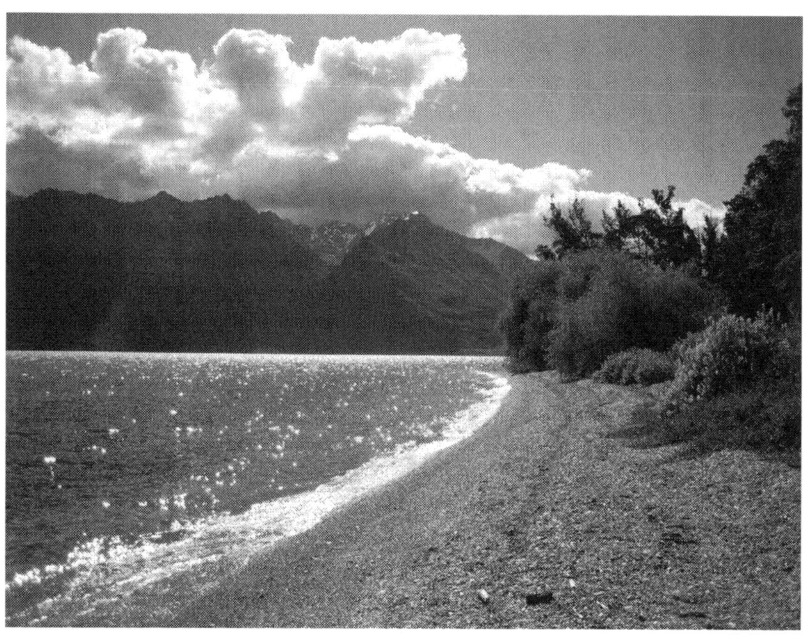

Actions Summary

Step 1: Obtain a doctor's prescription for pancreatic enzyme replacement pills to use with all meals and snacks.

Step 2: Complete the crucial EPI medical exams to help with the diagnosis, including a nutrition organic acid test, an MRCP MRI scan, comprehensive stool and blood tests.

Step 3: Be strict with food and water quality, including only eating non-processed, primal, organic (Bio in Europe) food.

Step 4: Rebalance nutrient deficiencies, including macronutrients, micronutrients, phytonutrients, fatty acids, and amino acids.

Step 5: Check for small intestinal bacterial overgrowth and perform the SIBO healing actions, if present.

Step 6: Check for Candida yeast overgrowth and perform the Candida healing actions, if present.

Step 7: Be strict and resolve silent or acid reflux, if present.

Step 8: Work on microbiome dysbiosis rebalancing.

Step 9: Work on actions to reduce oxidative stress, inflammation, and any insults to the body in your control.

Step 10: Work on neurotransmitter rebalancing.

Step 11: Utilize other primal healing elements in order to help your body in the healing process.

The good news is that there is hope! I was able to go from being bedridden and homebound for years with no glimmer of any future to enjoying life again. In this chapter I summarize the concrete actions that you can consider to help turn your health, or lack thereof, in a better direction. These steps are particularly useful to those with pancreas damage like pre- or full-blown exocrine pancreatic insufficiency. However, also sufferers of ME/CFS or other chronic ailments can benefit from many of these actions. Many actions are transferable to any type of healing, anti-aging or health maintenance. Hopefully doctors reading this can consider many of the steps to help patients with similar symptoms.

It is not a quick and easy fix, and it requires discipline and perseverance, which you have just by the fact that you are still reading this book. Once you tackle a few key elements, you will start to reduce the overall negative burden to your body. You will create a better environment from which to try to heal and slowly work on all the various related health issues.

Some symptoms can be resolved quickly by fixing nutrient deficiencies, but others take some time. Because your whole system potentially needs to be helped back into balance, and many areas are interlinked, there are a few key elements that need immediate attention. The actions are loosely listed in order of importance from my experience, but with benefit of hindsight many can be done in parallel.

It is tough to maintain a positive mindset if you have been feeling ill for such a long time, with no end in sight. During the healing process, try to hold on to any little improvement, and be grateful to yourself for having the determination to continue pushing through. Also have someone remind you how bad things were a month, a year, two years ago, etc. as it can be easy to forget when you are improving slowly. Tackle those few things that you do have control over and be determined. Keep an end goal in mind and ask yourself why you want to be healthier again. My stubbornness and wanting to see myself on a surfboard again, or be strong enough to be able to go on a walk with my wife again helped get me through the stages of disbelief, fear, anger, sadness, and acceptance throughout the healing process.

In the end you are your own best health advocate. No doctor, family member or friend will care or understand as much as you do about your own health. I had to do the research and study as if my life depended on it, which it did. Few doctors will have read more on your specific topic than you, because their interest and time availability for your case is not at the same survival level. Once you accept these things you can get to work. Please don't give up or become disillusioned during the process!

This recovery process is where patience and the strength of will comes into play, as it can take a while to start healing all the areas that were damaged over time. Your body will have begged, borrowed and stolen nutrients from wherever it could, just to keep the heart beating or the brain synapsis firing, as it tries very hard to keep you alive. During the suffering period you are essentially using your own muscle and bone for nutrient fuel in order to stay alive. In the meantime nothing heals, your immune system and organs slowly start sputtering, mitochondria start to dysfunction and die off, etc. One doctor mentioned that however long the decline was, that is likely how long it would take to recover. Hopefully by sharing my experiences it can help others with a similar issue recover far more quickly than that.

Of course, with anything you read in books and on the internet, this is just my personal experience. Do your homework, talk to your doctors and similar sufferers, be skeptical, and think things through for your personal situation and specific needs.

The chapter is broken down into the following eleven sections to start you on the path to better health:

1. Pancreatic enzyme replacement therapy (PERT).

2. Crucial EPI testing.

3. Food and water quality improvements.

4. Nutrient deficiencies rebalancing, and supplements.

5. Small intestinal bacterial overgrowth rebalancing.

6. Candida yeast overgrowth rebalancing.

7. Silent or acid reflux rebalancing.

8. Microbiome dysbiosis rebalancing.

9. Oxidative stress, bodily insults and inflammation reduction.

10. Neurotransmitters rebalancing.

11. Other primal healing elements.

1. Pancreatic Enzyme Replacement

The most important medicine to get immediately if you have any level of exocrine pancreatic insufficiency (EPI) is pancreatic enzyme replacement, also known as pancrelipase. If there is even a suspicion which has not been diagnosed yet, discuss a prescription with your doctor instead of having to potentially wait weeks for tests and results. Pancreatic enzyme replacement therapy (PERT) pills keep me alive, by allowing food and beverage intake to be broken down into their useful nutrient pieces and be absorbed. It impacts all deficiencies as well as calorie absorption.

Figure out the dosage you need per meal and know how to spread the pills during the meal. Do not go for non-prescription or vegetarian, unless as an additional supplement. Knowing the units to take per meal, with the peace of mind that the pill's strength is tightly controlled, is vital for your health.

Without this medicine you will continue in a vicious cycle where the pancreas does not produce enough enzymes, you do not get enough nutrients, and the pancreas as well as the rest of your body continue to break down. Luckily there are a few options available nowadays with different ratios of lipase (breaks down fats), protease (breaks down proteins), and amylase (breaks down carbohydrates). A healthy pancreas produces adequate quantities of these enzymes at the right time, and delivers them to the duodenum through the pancreatic ducts, in order to break down fats, proteins, and carbohydrates into usable nutrients. A few points to note:

- **Pancrelipase**: This is the generic term for the pancreatic enzymes mixture containing lipase, protease, and amylase. Pancrelipase prescription medicine is used to provide these enzymes.

- Start with enteric-coated (a.k.a. delayed release) pills so that it survives the passage through the acid bath in the stomach to the duodenum, where it is needed to break down your food. Discuss with your doctor if there is any specific reason why you would need a non-enteric coated version, which will need to be taken along with a stomach acid reducer.

• Some of the most well-known brands of pancrelipase are: Creon, Pancreaze, Ultresa, Viokace (not enteric coated), Pertzye and Zenpep.

• Choose one brand and stick with it for a while so your body can get accustomed to it. You can then determine the optimal amount per meal and snack without changing the variable of the pill brand and content. Get a prescription for all sizes, so you can build up a few months buffer and not have to worry about running out.

• For every person the optimal dosage varies based on your pancreas function, the type, fat content, and size of the meal. Experiment with the quantities to see what works for you. It can also change over time, so you will have to monitor your symptoms, such as stool quality and nutrient deficiencies.

• If you are taking too little you will notice your stool get smellier, skinnier, softer or yellower. It will also affect your nutrient levels, and after a while some of the symptoms.

• If you are taking too much you can get gastritis, burning, or acid pain type feeling in the stomach, and even slight nausea.

• After you have set a baseline amount per meal, experiment with increasing or decreasing increments of 12,000 lipase units until you are happy.

• Depending on the severity of your pancreas damage and EPI, even with PERT, food absorption is still likely not going to be the same as someone with a completely healthy pancreas. You will have to figure out through trial and error what is the optimal quantity to take with each meal or snack.

- Take the pills with every single meal, snack, or drink with calories (no need with plain water, coffee or tea) in order to break it down into usable nutrients.

- It is important to spread the pills throughout the meal. If I take three pills, I take the first pill after the first bite, the next somewhere in the middle of the meal, and the last pill about 80-90% through the meal.

- High protease content pancrelipase may be more helpful in reducing pain. This is likely due to breaking down more protein into the amino acids needed when deficient in certain neurotransmitters. Pancrelipase with high lipase content may be more effective in patients with steatorrhea, by breaking down more fat. This is just part of the personal adjustments of the quantities and type of enzyme pill you choose. It was not a big deciding factor for me, as I just take more pills when I eat a larger or richer meal.

- Dosages per pill are noted by their lipase enzyme content. For example, a Creon 36,000 USP pill contains at least 36,000 units of lipase, but also contains 114,000 units of protease and 180,000 units of amylase.

This website explains the workings of PERT quite well:

- https://www.creon.com/how-creon-works

Standard dosage guidelines are as follows:

Initial: 500 lipase units per kilogram of body weight per meal.

Maintenance: 400 to 2,500 lipase units per kilogram of body weight per meal.

Maximum: 10,000 lipase units per kilogram of body weight per day.

For snacks, depending on the size of the snack of course, use about half the dosage of a meal. You will fine tune it over time.

For example, for an 80 kg (176 Lbs.) person:

• Initial per meal would be 40,000 lipase units.

• Maintenance would be between 32,000 and 200,000 lipase units per meal.

• Maximum would be 800,000 lipase units per day.

As recently as 2009, Creon was approved by the FDA as the first dosage controlled pancreatic enzyme pill, but generic pancrelipase has been around for over a hundred years. Sales in prescription pancrelipase have drastically increased in the last few years, which give an indication of how many people are struggling with this issue. You can buy over-the-counter vegetarian or health food store versions whilst you wait to get your doctor's prescription. But, they are not going to give you the accurate and steady amounts you need to improve your health in a controlled manner. You can use them in addition to, but not in lieu of prescription versions.

As a little side note, because I was nauseous on and off for about six months, and every meal was torture, my doctor prescribed the following anti-nausea medicines to help take the edge off along with PERT:

• **Ondansetron, Promethazine**: Both are prescription anti-nausea medicine, which I only used during the really rough weeks when it was tough to keep food down.

2. Crucial EPI Testing

In Chapter 4 I covered the five crucial EPI tests in detail, as well as quite a few other tests that are very useful in checking for underlying issues, related health effects, nutrient deficiencies, tracking improvements as well as routine maintenance. These five tests should be considered at a minimum in order to diagnose pancreas damage and exocrine pancreatic insufficiency (EPI). They could also potentially provide an answer as to why you have been suffering from a wide variety of symptoms, including ME/CFS.

1. MRI of the Abdomen with MRCP Sequence

It was the most important test for me in spotting the advanced fatty atrophy of the pancreas. It also provides great information on liver, stomach, pancreas, pancreatic ducts, gallbladder and intestines. Ask for the MRCP (Magnetic Resonance Cholangiopancreatography) sequence, with and without contrast for better detail.

2. Nutritional Organic Acids Test (OAT)

This is an amazing test that can not only benefit those with suspected pancreas damage, but also those with ME/CFS, or any chronic or unexplained health issues. In my case it showed all of the following issues even before EPI was officially diagnosed:

- Pancreatic enzyme issues.
- Malabsorption and intestinal dysbiosis.
- Mitochondrial dysfunction.
- Candida yeast overgrowth.
- Small intestinal bacterial overgrowth (SIBO).
- Nutrient deficiencies in specific vitamins, minerals, fatty acids, and amino acids.
- Neurotransmitter issues.
- Oxidative stress issues.

Either or both are great as they provide slightly different takes. The Genova test now has an add-on section on essential and metabolic fatty acids, and provides some toxic metal and essential minerals levels. I prefer to do the plasma amino acids version instead of urine as I have read it is more accurate.

- **Genova Diagnostics**

NutrEval FMV or ONE (Optimal Nutritional Evaluation) FMV

- **The Great Plains Laboratory**

Nutritional and Metabolic Profile

3. Comprehensive Stool Analysis with Elastase.

Either of the following two tests provides a valuable picture of your intestinal health. I still do either one of them occasionally to make sure I am staying on track.

- **Doctor's Data**

Comprehensive Stool Analysis / Parasitology.

- **Genova Diagnostics**

Comprehensive Digestive Stool Analysis 2.0 with Fecal Fat Distribution.

One additional confirmation of EPI on this test is the pancreatic elastase element. If elastase shows the slightest bit under the threshold value of 200 (µg/mL), consider taking pancreatic enzymes, as well as performing further tests. Another good indicator of malabsorption which can point to EPI is the analysis of short chain fatty acids (SCFA) that these stool tests provide.

4. 24 Hour Fecal Lipids test

This test checks how much undigested fat is in your stool. To be even more accurate you can do a seventy-two hour collection, but I only did the twenty-four hour test. With EPI the pancreas is not producing enough enzymes to break down fat properly and thus lipids will be elevated in your stool. Please note, it does not have to be elevated much to be an indication of an issue.

5. 13C Mixed Triglyceride (MTG) Breath Test

It is a non-invasive way to test pancreatic lipase activity, i.e., fat digestion in the duodenum. It takes four to six hours in a specialized facility. It is considered a bit more accurate than the elastase test for moderate EPI. Since my doctor had already established EPI with the other tests, this one I did not do as it would have been superfluous. But if the elastase test did not confirm it for you, this can be one to consider.

Endocrine Pancreas Attention

As an important side note, since pre- and full-blown diabetes can be linked with EPI, it is also crucial to tackle the endocrine side. Consider these tests as well:

- **Hemoglobin A1c** (HbA1c)
- **Insulin** and **C-peptide**
- **Fasting glucose**

There are more details on these in Chapter 4. They are an easy way to determine if your sugar and carb intake is too high. In addition, the following hints from your body will indicate if your sugar and carb consumption is too high. When you have:

- Difficulty eating your daily food within a ten to twelve hours window.

- Nightly cravings, or feel the need to constantly snack.

- Hypoglycemic episodes.

- "Hangry" (hungry and angry) episodes, which means you are unable to efficiently use your own fat as fuel. Sugar is addictive, and this is a type of withdrawal symptom.

3. Food and Water Quality

This action is an absolute must in order to help your body heal! Consider the steps outlined in Chapter 6 for pancreas damage healing. If you also suffer from small intestinal bowel or Candida yeast overgrowth, or are hampered by acid or silent reflux, also consider the food actions in Chapter 7.

The key is to be very strict during the initial reset of your diet, for two to three months. When symptoms, sensitivities and blood test results start to improve, you can slowly reintroduce certain healthy food items. But pay close attention to how your body reacts and feels, and reintroduce just one item at a time in a controlled manner. The great thing is that the awareness and selection of healthy, organic (Bio or biological in Europe) food in supermarkets has increased tremendously.

Some food and water related changes will be beneficial for the rest of your life, but others can be temporary during the healing period. This is an area over which you have complete control in order to improve and maintain your quality of life.

Your body will thank you.

4. Nutrient Deficiencies and Supplements

The following areas all need to be considered, and supplements can be very important in the healing process:

• **Macronutrients**
Calories for energy through carbohydrates, proteins, and fats.

• **Micronutrients**
Vitamins, minerals, trace elements.

• **Phytonutrients**
Plant based chemicals such as carotenoids or flavonoids.

• **Fatty Acids**:
Essential omega-3, -6, and nonessential omega-9.

• **Amino Acids**:
Essential and nonessential building blocks of protein.

You often hear the advice to get your nutrients through balanced and varied food, and not supplements. That is great if you are able to get all the necessary nutrients each day through high quality food, which was grown in an herbicide and pesticide free environment, in nutrient rich soil. However, this is just not realistic even if you are seemingly completely healthy. The high paced lifestyles, daily stress, toxic environmental load, lack of time and effort spent on quality food purchasing and preparation, difficulty and expense in getting quality fresh organic food, modern agricultural practices, depleted soil, etc. make it very difficult.

Your food will likely not contain all the necessary nutrients at optimal levels each and every day. In addition, if you are suffering from any pancreas damage, nutritional deficiencies, malabsorption, SIBO, Candida, microbiome dysbiosis, oxidative stress, any illness, or are taking medicines, this advice is not helpful either. If you are ill, your body requires far more of a specific nutrient than you would be able to get from eating a balanced diet. If you are older, your absorption, intestinal, pancreatic and metabolic functions are just not as efficient and effective as before. With EPI you are already deficient. You just cannot eat enough of a particular food type to get the nutrient amounts required to get all your metabolic pathways back to functioning optimally, and heal some of your resultant symptoms.

All this then lands you in a vicious cycle, making you get worse over time. People with EPI are the perfect Petri dish for testing the effectiveness of supplements, and I can tell you from personal experience that I would not be here today if not for their availability. The other thing you hear often, even from doctors, is that supplements have not been proven to make a difference. But again, this is made with the assumption that you are completely healthy, and you would not be talking to the doctor if you were. Also, women are advised to take additional supplements during pregnancy, so how is that any different from someone who needs additional supplementation due to illness, aging, or deficiencies?

Some terms you hear these days are bio-hacking, life-extension or anti-aging therapies, many of which fall back on the power of nutrients on the body. EPI is quite the opposite. It is akin to being a pro-aging or an anti-life extension therapy due to the lack of nutrients. This hinders the efficiency and efficacy of metabolic pathways, with subsequent rapid aging effects. As with anything you read these days, check credentials, wonder about monetary motivations, be critical, skeptical and hold on to your common sense when reading about or buying supplements. There is a lot of quackery and greedy monetary motivation out there, which sadly creates more noise you do not need. But please do not outrightly dismiss this important healing avenue. Please consider the following actions:

Step 1. Take the Nutrition Status Tests

A few simple tests, including the nutritional organic acid and Spectracell tests I mentioned previously can provide a baseline check for deficiencies, and subsequently allow you to see how well you are recovering. The better you get and feel, the less frequently you will need to take them. Chapter 4 contains the details on many more valuable additional health tests which were helpful to me and might be of interest to you as well.

Step 2. Take Supplements

Chapter 5 is quite detailed in all the areas of supplementation to consider, and is logically laid out by area of concern. Not only does it list supplements for deficiencies, but also to potentially support related problem areas such as SIBO, Candida, mitochondrial dysfunction, and microbiome dysbiosis. Supplements that helped me are listed in the following categories:

- Amino acids

- Antioxidant support
- EPI
- Intestinal healing
- Methylation
- Mitochondrial (also for CFS)
- Neurotransmitter
- Omega-3
- SIBO, Candida yeast overgrowth
- Vitamins and minerals

Examples of Supplementation Success

Throughout the book I have mentioned examples of what are really just classic biochemistry in practice, and areas where supplements have helped me. Below are a few examples:

- If you have insufficient levels of vitamin B6 or copper, your metabolic pathways can struggle to produce enough neurotransmitters, with subsequent depression or chronic pain as a result.

- If you have insufficient amino acids glutamine, glycine and cysteine along with vitamins B1, B2, B6, and B12, magnesium, and zinc you can have trouble producing a key antioxidant glutathione, with subsequent oxidative stress, mitochondrial dysfunction, and ATP production issues.

- Testosterone production requires, for example, vitamins B6, B9, C, D, E, K, zinc, magnesium, and carnitine. My low levels increased by 80% and were resolved without testosterone replacement hormones, but just by resolving nutrient deficiencies.

- My asthma-like breathing issues, heart rhythm issues, shortness of breath, paresthesia, panic attacks, anxiety in the pit of my stomach, inability to sleep, blood pressure spikes, coordination issues, to name a few, were all resolved with the help of supplements such as magnesium, CoQ10, carnitine and B vitamins.

- My easy bruising was resolved by vitamin K2 supplements.

- Consider an amino acid supplement for pain reduction. Almost all the amino acids are necessary to produce endorphins, the body's natural painkiller, so if you lack just one you cannot produce endorphins properly. It helped me to avoid hardcore and addicting painkillers like opioids.

Deficiencies in Macronutrients

Often with EPI you have lost muscle weight and thus supplementing macronutrients in the form of, for example, medical food can help. This is a powder or shake that includes extra calories from healthy organic carbohydrates, protein and fats. These medical food supplements usually also includes a long list of micronutrients and phytonutrients.

Deficiencies in Micronutrients and Phytonutrients

Micronutrients and phytonutrients come in many different forms, both individually or as part of a multi-vitamin, multi-mineral, or a pill with multiple ingredients addressing a specific area of support.

Something to consider is a reputable doctor or clinic where you can get vitamin and mineral drips or injections. Interestingly, I stumbled across this suggestion by reading EPI information for dogs by veterinarians. It is also where I read that 80% of dogs with EPI also suffer from SIBO. Functional or integrative medicine doctors often have this service as part of their practice. It is a way to avoid the intestinal system, bypass malabsorption issues, and get them straight into the bloodstream. Magnesium, B complex, and C are quite standard. Glutathione antioxidant is another you can get through a drip, however, this caused cracking headaches in my case. Not everyone has issues with the glutamate component in glutathione, which is similar to having an MSG sensitivity, but just be aware of it.

If you are not already using one, I would immediately start with a daily, high quality, multi-vitamins and multi-minerals pill. But, depending on your deficiencies, this will likely not be sufficient initially.

Since EPI sufferers have a hard time breaking down fat, the fat-soluble nutrients can be deficient, including A, D, E and K, and the often overlooked but crucial coenzyme CoQ10.

Mitochondrial support supplements are also an important consideration because ME/CFS is nasty and can last a long time. I had breathing and heart issues due to secondary mitochondrial dysfunction which was caused by nutrient deficiencies. The symptoms were resolved with supplements like L-carnitine, CoQ10, vitamins B1, B2, creatine, D-ribose, nicotinamide riboside, MitoThera, CorvalenM and ATP Fuel.

Deficiencies in Fatty Acids

The idea that you should eat less fat when you have pancreatic damage or suffer from EPI is old-fashioned thinking, and hinders your healing process. You likely need more essential fatty acids initially in order to heal, than even a healthy person. The issue with EPI is that you are unable to break down fats and absorb essential fatty acids without PERT. They are essential because your body cannot produce them, but we need them for healthy cell walls, mitochondrial function, and to survive. Along with pancreatic enzymes pills and adjusting your food, you can supplement essential fatty acids with a few simple actions. Test your levels with for example the Genova Diagnostics's FMV test, which has an add-on option that details your fatty acid levels.

The three fatty acid "supplementations" I have taken, with pancreatic enzymes of course, were mostly through my food and all in moderation:

- **Fish oil** (Omega-3): pills in glass bottles and small fish.
- **Coconut oil**: glass bottle organic version, and only temporarily.
- **Olive oil** (Omega-9): extra virgin, in glass bottles, with food.

Since we usually get plenty of the essential Omega-6, I did not supplement them except through seeds and nuts. As with anything, do not go extreme and test your levels for improvements or excess.

Deficiencies in Amino Acids

Amino acids are another crucial element that is often overlooked. Pancreatic enzymes are necessary to break down proteins into amino acids, and so people with EPI will likely have deficiencies. Even with pancreatic enzyme replacement I still need to supplement amino acids. Amino acid supplements can be taken without needing to take enzymes, since they are already broken down from proteins. I was taking a multi-amino acid supplement which includes all the twenty main amino acids, multiple times per day for many months, but am now down to just sporadic use. If I feel muscle pain waking up, especially in my thighs, it is a sign that I need to supplement.

What I did not know is that animals, including ourselves and the animals we eat, are unable to produce the nine essential amino acids. Only plants, fungus and bacteria can do this for us. This is another reason that balancing your microbiome, avoiding chlorinated water, and eating only organic is so important. We need to take in these essential amino acids and absorb them every day. We cannot store them except as our own muscle tissue, which will be used as protein fuel for the body if deficient.

Actions to take

There are two amino acid supplements which I still use today.

- **Amino acid complex.** A pill containing the essential (we are unable to make them in the body) and nonessential (we are able to make them if we have sufficient cofactors) amino acids. During the healing months I took a pill one to three times per day, thirty minutes prior to my meal. Now I still use it sporadically. No PERT is needed with these.

- **Organic** (Bio in Europe) **vegan** or **single ingredient whey protein powders.** You want an organic only product where you trust the source and country of origin of the ingredients used, without sugars, artificial flavors and sugars, preservatives, or other chemicals added. To skip a transfer process you can use vegan instead of animal based, because only plants are able to produce the essential amino acids. Mix it up a bit based on the amino acid content, your taste (e.g., rice, pea, hemp) and any sensitivities you might have. I had trouble with too much pea content, for example. Be careful with soy based ones; I avoid them myself. To get an indication of the amount of essential amino acids to eat you can use the calculation table from the World Health Organization, which is in Chapter 5. Keep in mind that you do need pancreatic enzymes to break down protein powder into usable amino acids.

As with everything, do not go extreme, as when proteins are digested the body becomes more acidic (hence amino acid). Your kidneys work hard to regulate acidity, but if the acidity is too high your body can pull calcium from your bones to offset this. Too much protein will also turn into glucose through the gluconeogenesis pathway. Excess amino acids in urine, abnormal urea nitrogen (BUN test), or ammonia levels in the blood can all indicate issues with excess protein. As a guideline the RDA and WHO recommend around 0.8 grams of protein per kilogram of body weight if you are sedentary. The paleo community recommends around 1.5 grams per kilogram of lean body weight for active people. I eat somewhere in between. During healing periods, high physical activity, and muscle building you will need more than if you are maintaining or sedentary.

Supplementing with amino acids was a key piece in the healing puzzle and it helped me in areas such as:

- Muscle loss. I no longer had painful muscles waking up in the morning, as my body no longer needed to cannibalize my own muscle for protein.
- Depression, apathy and mood.
- Pain and malaise.
- Chronic fatigue.

5. Small Intestinal Bacterial Overgrowth

This is one of the areas that I wish I had known about a lot earlier, as it impedes healing and causes malabsorption as well as a whole host of other symptoms. If you suffer from SIBO, or suspect that you do, please follow the steps in Chapter 7 to help diagnose and rebalance. It is likely that you are suffering from this if you have any pancreatic damage, or even if you have been on a standard modern Western diet.

6. Candida Yeast Overgrowth

If you suffer from yeast overgrowth, or suspect that you do, please follow the steps in Chapter 7 to help diagnose and rebalance. If you have not been breaking down food properly due to lack of pancreatic enzymes, it is likely that the fungi in your system will be out of balance and have flourished in places where they should not have.

7. Silent or Acid Reflux

If you suffer from acid or silent reflux, or suspect that you do, please follow the steps in Chapter 7 to tackle it, which includes:

1. Raising the head of your bed.
2. SIBO and Candida actions.
3. Top-down acid reduction, including temporary diet.
4. Bottom-up acid reduction.

It is likely that you are suffering from this if you have any pancreatic damage, or even if you have been on a standard modern Western diet.

Whether it is the overt pain after eating or drinking version, or the silent reflux version, this is a symptom that needs to be resolved by diet and not constant symptom suppressing drugs like acid reducers or proton pump inhibitors. Acid reflux is your body telling you something is wrong with your food and beverage intake, as well as signaling dysbiosis in your stomach and intestines.

8. Microbiome Dysbiosis

In Chapter 3 microbiome imbalance causes and effects were discussed, but what can you do about it?

Step 1. Perform tests

A few simple tests worth taking can provide helpful information on intestinal dysbiosis and help track improvements. Pick at least one nutrition, and one stool test. These are the ones I have taken:

• **Doctor's Data**
Comprehensive Stool Analysis / Parasitology.

• **Genova Diagnostics**
Comprehensive Digestive Stool Analysis 2.0 with Fecal Fat Distribution.

• **Genova Diagnostics**
NutrEval FMV or ONE (Optimal Nutritional Evaluation) FMV

• **Great Plains Lab**
Nutritional and Metabolic Profile Organic Acid.

Step 2. Rebalancing Actions

• Evaluate and resolve any SIBO or Candida yeast overgrowth.

• Reevaluate your food and water quality consumption.

• Add probiotics supplements. It is an area that is still not understood well, and there are some studies which show that it has little effectiveness, but I have had good luck with some. But, I only use the refrigerated kinds which are quite expensive. Use 10-

15 billion units or more, as anything less will likely not make it past your stomach acid.

• Add prebiotics. Non-digestible fiber that is food for bacteria. It is best taken in through food, e.g., garlic, artichoke, leek, onions, jicama root, asparagus, or green banana. Also include fermented products like sauerkraut, kimchee, natto, atjar, miso, or tempeh.

• Look at unsweetened, fermented, full fat dairy with live bacteria cultures like yoghurt, Kefir or buttermilk.

• Stop using antibacterial soaps, sprays, detergents, toothpaste and mouthwash (good bacteria in your mouth are important too) in your home. Of course cleaning is very important, but there are many other options beside products containing antibiotics.

• Improve water quality and avoid anything with added chlorine, chloramine or fluorides.

• Eat organic in order to lower the constant exposure to synthetic herbicides, pesticides and antibiotics. It is used on almost everything, including animal feed and thus any animal products.

• Drastically lower sugar and processed carbs. Aim your HbA1c, a multi-week marker of blood glucose, to be 5.2% or below.

• Be careful with antibiotics courses and ointments, and only take them if absolutely necessary. Replenish the good bacteria immediately during the course with pre- and probiotics, as you do not want the "empty real estate" left by the antibiotics "cluster bomb" to be filled with dysbiotic bacteria.

• Fecal Microbiota Transplant (FMT), which is invasive and I have not tried it, is where fecal matter from a healthy person is transplanted to help heal the microbiome. This I read is only for extreme cases and, e.g., C. difficile colitis bacterial overgrowth.

Perhaps in the future there will be a method whereby probiotics are tailor-made for each individual. Ones that after a simple test can combine where you live, your diet, where and how you were born, and any deficiencies, in order to determine the optimal levels and types of bacteria to put in the pill. A pill designed to be the perfect delivery system, which deposits the probiotics to just the right place in your intestines.

I am still waiting for the science fiction scene to become reality where, after your morning toilet visit, any micronutrient deficiencies or microbiome imbalances are measured from your urine and stool. Then, from the analysis immediately following, a 3D printer creates your daily health balancing micronutrient pill.

9. Oxidative Stress, Insults and Inflammation

Stemming as many insults to the body as you can, and supporting your antioxidant system, can help heal the body, improve mitochondrial health, reduce systemic inflammation, and lower oxidative stress. Oxidative stress, simplistically the rusting damage inside the body, is a major cause of health breakdowns. I cannot stress enough how important a factor this is to address, in order to reduce further damage and help the body to heal. Inadequate antioxidant function can cause mitochondrial damage and pancreatic acinar cell atrophy.

Inflammation is really a combination of elements, but I want to specifically mention it since it is so important to overall healing. Few doctors will discuss root cause or practical steps to take, unless to prescribe some drugs. Of course inflammation is the body's reaction to fix a problem, whether it is an invader like a pathogen (e.g., bacteria, virus, or fungus), or even a perceived invader (e.g., gluten) in an autoimmune type reaction, or a wound. But due to the constant bombardment of chemicals and toxins in our water, excessive sugar, pesticides and herbicides in the food, and an imbalanced microbiome, the body can be in a constant state of inflammation. This requires a tremendous amount of energy and nutrients, which people with EPI, CFS, or other illnesses do not have to spare. Inflammation also decreases tryptophan and serotonin levels. To bring this systemic inflammation down, you first have to eliminate or reduce as many of the health aggravations as you can.

Pancreas damage and intestinal inflammation can really hurt. A common path taken by some doctors is painkillers, since investigating the source of pain and inflammation is time consuming and difficult. Of course, in many situations the pain can be too much and may really require pain medication. However, in my case I did not want to become addicted to painkillers, and even something as simple as Ibuprofen would make me feel worse. Pain is a signal from the body that something is wrong and you need to heal. Painkillers do not resolve the root cause, but mask this signal. So instead I followed the steps outlined in this book. Swelling, inflammation and pain were lowered, and even something as seemingly unrelated as deep molar pain, for which the dentist recommended a root canal, completely went away when my systemic inflammation was lowered.

Below are a few actions, in no specific order, which you can take to assist your body in trying to get back in balance.

Step 1. Lower Insults to Your Body

When your body is constantly burning through energy and nutrients due to systemic inflammation and a high burden of toxic insults it needs to clean out of the system, it makes it tough to heal and feel better. At this stage you have to be frugal with your energy allocation, and not unnecessarily waste energy when it can be avoided. Anything that you are exposed to that is not a nutrient needs to be filtered out of your body, costing precious nutrients and taxing the antioxidant processes.

- Reduce exposure to viruses, bacteria, and fungus as much as possible. This means avoiding sick people and areas where there is much potential exposure. Use surgical masks if need be. Do not be afraid, out of politeness, to sit somewhere away from an overtly sick, snottery or coughing person. Be especially careful if you have to travel in an airplane, or public transportation, are in a children's playground or daycare facility, or if you have to go to a hospital or doctor's office. And of course the obvious actions, such as washing and drying of hands, being cautious about shaking of hands or kissing as a greeting, or touching your face with your hands, etc.

• Avoid any foods or substances that you are sensitive or allergic to. I had mentioned one such sensitivity and allergy test in Chapter 4, which might give a good indication.

• Avoid smoking (even secondary), alcohol, and recreational drugs.

• Reduce chemical exposure. This could be from so many sources, including in your home, at work, from packaged or non-organic food, tap water, packaging materials, cleaning supplies, dishwashing soap, washing detergents, carpet cleaners, toothpaste, herbicides, pesticides, fumigation materials, cosmetics, hair products, deodorant, sunscreen lotion, perfumes, etc.

• Reduce toxic heavy metal exposure. For example, avoid heavy industrial areas, be careful when filling up your car since gasoline has additives like thallium in it, careful with fresh paint, and avoid construction or demolition areas. When you feel strong enough consider a qualified dentist who can safely replace any metal amalgam fillings which include mercury. Choose a dentist who understands the importance of using air filtration and metal ingestion avoidance during the process.

• In Chapter 4 I listed a few tests that were helpful in determining levels of toxic metals and chemicals in the body. These are good indicators of trouble spots causing your body to be in a constant high state of detoxification and inflammatory stress.

• Avoid sunscreens that contain substances like benzophenone, oxybenzone, or 4-methylbenzylidene camphor.

• Reduce plastics and styrofoam exposure, including food cans (lining), plastic water bottles, soda cans (lining) and bottles, milk cartons (lining), fast food wrappers, red party cups, to-go drink and coffee cups, to-go boxes, straws, food storage containers, plastic water boilers, plastic cooking wares, microwave meal dishes, etc. Replace your plastic containers, cups and plates at home with glass such as Pyrex or porcelain. Replace your plastic water boiler with a glass or lead free metal one. BPA is still used a lot, however, this is not the only chemical that is leached into your food and drinks from plastic exposure. Phthalates, BPF, BPS and PFCs are other good examples. Small plastic particles are found in unfiltered tap water and all plastic water bottles. It is impossible to avoid plastics completely, but reduce exposure wherever possible.

• Avoid unfiltered North American tap water and ice cubes due to the toxins and heavy metals not filtered out adequately, and the added chlorine, chloramine and fluoride. Micro-plastic contamination is another big problem. Depending on where you live, check your water supply quality, or pay for a clean water delivery service.

• Take a good look at prescription drugs, pain pills and their possible side effects. Check with your doctor if you really need to take them all, or if you have gone into a vicious cycle where one medicine is to fix the symptoms caused by another medicine.

• Improve your sleep hygiene and take naps. Sleep heals!

• Avoid stressful people, situations, blogs, radio and TV programs, especially news (cannot do anything about it anyway) or the soapbox opinion shouting "news" programs.

• Avoid toxic people and those that leach energy from you, or make you emotional, if possible. Instead, surround yourself with understanding and supportive people as much as you can.

• Make your immediate environment and the area where you spend most of your time healing as cozy, comfortable and relaxed as possible.

• Reduce exposure to mold. If you suspect any areas of mold, have it checked by a professional. These companies can check your house for air quality and EMF exposure too.

• Lower your exposure to air pollutants by getting a quality air filter with at least a HEPA filter, and a sensor providing real-time air quality measurements. This pollution would include smog, dust, pet dander, mold, pollen, dust mites, volatile organic compounds (VOC), chemicals from carpet and furniture, gas stove, and other particles that you breathe in. If you live near an airport, busy street, highway, construction zones, agriculture, manufacturing, mining, or heavy industry, having an air filter is very important. Polluted air causes oxidative stress and is linked to different types of cancer. Try to get your bedroom to <10-15 (μg/m3) for PM2.5 and PM10 before going to bed.

• Reduce your exposure to excessive noise. If you live near busy roads, freeways, wind turbines or airports, consider getting double or triple paned glass. Or get some quality earplugs so it does not interrupt your sleep.

• Reduce your exposure to strong or continuous EMF fields as much as possible.

• Get a carbon filter on your shower to avoid the chlorine fumes from hot tap water that has chlorine or chloramines added in.

• Avoid drinking water that is demineralized, distilled, or RO without essential minerals added back in.

• Only buy organic (Bio in Europe), including restaurant and packaged food. You need to bring down the level of pesticides and herbicides, not to mention eat food with more nutrients left in them. Glyphosate type herbicides are everywhere, and it leaches key nutrients from vegetables, plants and grains, the effect of which is in the animal feed as well as our food, not to mention the antibiotics effect it has on your microbiome. Other impactful herbicides to avoid are the commonly used 2,4D and atrazine.

Atrazine (illegal in the EU) is used on most non-organic corn in North America, and thus fed to all non-organic animals.

• NSAIDs (Nonsteroidal anti-inflammatory drugs). This is where a good conversation with your doctor is necessary. NSAIDs address symptoms and do little for the root cause issue. There is a reason why your body is inflamed. By not only ignoring this message but suppressing it, things can become worse, especially when you do not reduce the hits to the body causing the inflammation in the first place. Of course there are valid reasons and important times for a short application, when you have something acute, but for chronic issues this is a different story. They can also affect the stomach lining, and thus can impact malabsorption, ulcers, and sensitivities. This is the last thing an EPI sufferer needs. Interesting to note is that acetaminophen (Not considered an NSAID), did not provide me with the same side effects as ibuprofen did on the few occasions that I took it.

• Try going gluten-free for a couple of months. When your microbiome is imbalanced and your intestinal lining has been compromised, gluten can be seen as an invader and cause the immune system to react to it. Even when you do not have celiac disease, this is important. Once you have confirmed you do not have celiac disease, and things have stabilized, you can try to reintroduce organic whole-grain gluten products, but be very careful and really watch the signs your body gives you. If it gives you any type of adverse inflammatory effect, stop eating it.

• Reduce most grains for a couple of months. With EPI it is difficult to keep muscle weight on and get the amount of nutrients you need, that is why you need to be a little cautious with going full blown grain-free. Certainly non-organic grains are to be avoided, but a small sized portion of organic wild rice is fine, unless you are diabetic. Bake your own organic paleo bread or eat organic paleo pasta made from things like quinoa or lentils. There are luckily many options these days. Just as with gluten, you can experiment when your microbiome and health have improved. I notice inflammation signs quickly in the form of redness and swelling in the top of my fingers near the nail's matrix, intestinal bloating, or painful joints. Everyone of course has different reactions and tolerances.

• Reduce blue light exposure from electronics.

• Drastically reduce sugar and processed carbs intake in all its forms. It is a recurring theme in prior chapters since it is so vital.

• Consider the food actions in Chapter 7 to help lower inflammation and oxidative stress. Delve into the primal lifestyle.

Step 2. Support Your Antioxidant System

In addition to reducing the assaults your antioxidant system has to handle, you can reduce systemic inflammation and oxidative stress through food quality and supplements. In prior chapters I discussed food and water quality as well as the importance of supplements. Especially with pancreas damage and EPI, and its subsequent nutrient deficiencies and ill functioning metabolic pathways, to add supplements in order to support your antioxidant processes is important. A few to consider supplementing during the healing period are:

- Vitamin A, C and E
- CoQ10
- Beta-carotene
- Alpha-lipoic acid
- Glutathione
- Superoxide dismutase

Further in this chapter I also have a small section on the benefits of oxidative stress reduction through earthing or grounding to try.

10. Neurotransmitters

With EPI, CFS, SIBO, Candida, microbiome dysbiosis or other gastrointestinal ailments it can be expected that you will have some kind of neurotransmitter imbalance, whether it is serotonin, dopamine, adrenaline (a.k.a. epinephrine), noradrenaline (a.k.a.

norepinephrine), or melatonin. This can in turn cause a whole range of potential symptoms, such as low energy, sleeping issues, brain fog, mood swings, chronic pain, hormone imbalances, concentration problems, memory issues, inflammation, apathy, depression, etc. The long term inability to produce sufficient dopamine, coupled with long term insulin resistance, might even be linked to Alzheimer's.

For me this was one of the last symptoms to resolve because of the dual cause of depression, both physical and mental. Firstly, there is the purely physical cause of not being able to produce sufficient amounts of neurotransmitters due to nutrient deficiencies like vitamins, minerals and amino acids. Nutrients are needed to stay in mental balance as well as lower pain. The stress of the illness itself, both physically and emotionally can also cause an extra demand on neurotransmitters, and thus deplete them more quickly than normal. When you are unable to be as physically active as normal, this also dampens neurotransmitter production. Secondly, there is the mental side. The loss of your normal, pre-illness quality of life dents the psyche. The traumatic experience can cause grief, anger, sadness, depression and loss of hope.

These neurotransmitter imbalance symptoms need to be tackled in a two-pronged approach, both mentally and physically.

Step 1. Physical Actions

• The nutritional organic acid tests mentioned before give a good indication of which neurotransmitters are out of balance, and which nutrients you are deficient in. There are other neurotransmitter tests listed in Chapter 4 as well.

• Nutrient deficiencies need to be tackled to help your body be able to produce sufficient neurotransmitters.

• Walk as soon as you are able to, and as much as your body allows, but make sure to pace yourself to avoid setbacks; baby steps. Initially I had to start with just walking around the living room, or go up and down the stairs, before managing a very slow stroll to the end of the block. That was a big milestone.

• Later on, when you have recovered from much of the nutritional imbalances, and you are getting a little stronger, start with very small weights and some physiotherapy to step up physical activity. This stimulates production of neurotransmitters.

• The microbiome has a lot to do with imbalances. Clostridia bacteria, for example, can inhibit the transfer of dopamine to norepinephrine. Bifidobacteria produce folate (vitamin B9), which is needed in activities such as methylation. Chlorinated tap water, antibiotic treatments, herbicides and pesticides all help to imbalance your microbiome. Methylation is also involved in neurotransmitter production. Work on rebalancing your microbiome as outlined previously.

• Combining Betaine (a.k.a. TMG or Trimethylglycine) with SAMe (a source for methionine) has been demonstrated in research to help with depression.

Supplements can help. Consider them before any heavy antidepressants, which have their own side effect symptoms (ironically depression and suicide are some of them) and do not address any deficiency. I think that many people who are on prescription antidepressants these days are really suffering from microbiome dysbiosis, and nutrient deficiencies from the usual suspects of chlorinated tap water, excessive sugar, bad diets, and herbicide overexposure. Remember, companies cannot get a patent on a healthy diet, an amino acid, vitamin or mineral.

A few related nutrient details to keep in mind for mental healing:

• **Phenylalanine**. An essential amino acid needed to produce tyrosine. It cannot be produced by animals and must come from food. DLPA (DL-Phenylalanine) supplement helped me with chronic pain and emotional lability.

• **Tryptophan**. An essential amino acid needed to produce serotonin, which in turn is used to produce melatonin. It cannot be produced by animals and must come from food. 5-HTP as well as an amino acid multi supplement helped me with depression.

• **Tyrosine**. An amino acid needed to produce dopamine, which in turn is needed to produce norepinephrine. Neuro Balance, a supplement with tyrosine and vitamins B1, B2, and B6, helped me with fatigue, feelings of apathy, loss of life-joy, and the what's-the-point thoughts.

• **Tetrahydrobiopterin (BH4).** It is an essential cofactor required for the production of neurotransmitters dopamine, serotonin, melatonin, norepinephrine, and epinephrine. As a side note, it is also required for production of nitric oxide (NO). BH4 production requires the following cofactors:

• Vitamin C is required to recycle BH2 and BH3 into BH4.
• Molybdenum.
• Methyl folate, iron, vitamin B6, magnesium and copper.

• **GABA** (Gamma-aminobutyric acid), **taurine, inositol, and glycine.** They can all help your body naturally produce more of the calming neurotransmitters.

• **Anandamide.** It is a neurotransmitter and endocannabinoid produced in your brain that can help with pain and mood. Elements such as dark chocolate, exercise, kaempferol flavonoid containing foods, or cannabidiol (CBD) can help increase levels.

• **Serotonin.** For serotonin to be produced in the brain, tryptophan, vitamin D and omega-3 fatty acids are needed. It is the reason why taking vitamin D supplements quickly improved my mood, and provided more happier and optimistic thoughts. Serotonin provides a sense of well-being and reduces anxiety.

• **Melatonin** is a hormone which is synthesized from tryptophan. It is key in your sleep-wake (a.k.a. Circadian rhythm) cycle, by helping you fall and stay asleep. It follows the same metabolic pathway as serotonin, and thus needs vitamin B6, B9, B12, copper, zinc, and magnesium. Any deficiencies in those can cause sleep disruptions for which some doctors prescribe serious pharmaceuticals, as opposed to looking at a possible root cause. If you are having trouble sleeping, you can also consider a melatonin supplement temporarily.

As with all supplements, a bit of trial and error is needed for your situation.

Step 2. Mental Healing Actions

Anxiety, stress, sadness, loss of hope, depression, grief, apathy, anger, disappointment, resentment, fear are all part of the illness and healing process. It is a traumatic experience for which you will probably go through the usual rollercoaster process of denial, anger, bargaining, depression and acceptance. Sometimes it helps to talk with a professional like a psychiatrist, psychologist or therapist who is experienced with handling patients with chronic pain and illness. This is tough to do when you have so little energy for even a conversation with friends or family. But one of the goals is to learn some mental tools to cope a little better with your situation. Beware of those doctors that immediately want to prescribe you the standard antidepressant pills, as a considerable part of the cause of anxiety, depression and emotional lability with EPI is nutrient deficiency, and metabolic pathways that are not functioning properly.

But, even when the balance of nutrients has improved, there is a constant feeling of threat and dread of a relapse or setback. With days that can fluctuate wildly in malaise, pain and energy levels, keep reminding yourself that tomorrow could be a better day. In addition to seeking professional therapy, in the next section I outline one additional element which can help with the mental healing process, namely meditation, visualization, and imagery healing.

11. Other Primal Healing Elements

With the idea of every little bit helps, here are a few other elements that I incorporated during the healing period and beyond. The goal remains to lower the abuses to the body and provide a healing environment for the body and mind. Some have been around for thousands of years, and others may be a little unorthodox. Some ideas might seem a bit silly or controversial, but do not underestimate the power of placebo either. Your mind is quite powerful in its healing capacity. Some of these actions might not be an obvious part of the healing primal lifestyle. However, many of the environmental toxins, modern lifestyle pressures, and oxidative stress accelerators are a relatively recent phenomenon. Many of the healing elements have been around for a very long time. These are not in any particular order as they all can be helpful, some more than others, and they are not mutually exclusive.

1. Alternative Medicine

There is much controversy and noise surrounding some of the alternative medicine specialties. Of course, you have to do your due diligence to find well experienced, high quality, accredited practitioners, but to outright dismiss them would be a disservice to your healing process. Here are a few examples I looked into:

• **Naturopathy, Functional or Integrative Medicine**. It is often naturopaths, functional specialists, or integrative medicine specialists who have more knowledge and interest in the workings of metabolic pathways and supplements, and are able to order many non-standard tests like the nutrition organic acid tests. I had a really good integrative medicine doctor (an MD) who helped me with supplements as well as testing for a large range of deficiencies and symptoms. It is well worth finding a reputable, highly qualified doctor. Some also provide vitamin drips and injections as part of their service.

• **Massage, acupressure, neuromuscular therapy**. With all the layers of pain, and since my skin hurt for a long time, this was only possible for me at a later stage to help with relaxation, muscle and joint tightness. It is worth considering for blood circulation, muscle tenseness and de-stressing.

• **Acupuncture**. I tried many sessions prior to my diagnosis, but am not sure whether it helped me. In hindsight, I would not do it again before getting my pancreatic enzyme replacement therapy up and running, as well as a few nutrient deficiencies resolved. Because of my vitamin K deficiency at the time, it would often give me bruises as well. It is worth considering as I see how it can help with pain.

• **Energy Kinesiology.** This was a strange one as there was no physical touch and no machinery. I was quite skeptical and yet it unexplainably really gave me cracking headaches. Many others at the clinic were raving about how it helped them though.

• **Reiki**. A combination of massage and energy healing which has looked intriguing, but I never did end up trying it. It seems like it could help with relaxation.

• **Homeopathy**. This is one I would be careful with if suffering from EPI. Our immune system is already on edge, and struggling to function well due to the nutrient deficiencies. I did use a few botanicals during the Candida and SIBO treatment, but it was very specific to those issues. Homeopathy is simply taking in small quantities of substances to trigger the immune system, which may be more useful for other ailments.

• **Chiropractic**. Another one to be careful with. I did find a good, reputable sports medicine specialist who treats many professional athletes. But, I have also come across a few who were just in it for the money. Do not go to one who likes to crack you or perform fast twists of the neck, or who tells you that you need to come back every week for months at a time. If they start talking about payment plans, run! Not only is it not helpful, but this can be dangerous, especially when your musculoskeletal system has been weakened due to nutrient deficiencies with EPI.

• **Ayurveda and Chinese Herbology**. Respectively, ancient Indian and Chinese systems of medicine. The only elements I utilized were acupuncture, and some well-known spices (e.g., saffron, turmeric, ginger, fennel, black pepper, cinnamon, coriander, cloves). They have been around for thousands of years helping heal people, and they might be helpful to some.

2. Sauna

There are a few options I have tried, from Finnish, steam, far infra-red (FIR), and near infra-red (NIR). The goals are similar, increase blood circulation, improve circulation of the lymphatic system, sweat out toxins, and relax the body and mind. I tried both FIR and NIR sauna, but will stick with NIR sauna. The difference is in the frequency levels you are exposed to. FIR frequencies are much higher and will get you to sweat quicker. This might be helpful when going through a detoxing period and you want to sweat the toxins out of your skin quicker. However, many FIR setups are very high in electromagnetic (EMF) radiation, so you are likely doing more damage to your mitochondria and cells than the benefit. There are some low EMF FIR setups, so just be careful and check before usage. NIR can be done as easily as buying an inexpensive heat lamp setup, where you get the frequency spectrum that mimics the warming sun. Light waves of 600-950 (nm) can help your mitochondria. Just be careful to wear complete light blocking eye protection when using them. I prefer the personal sauna boxes where my head is not being heated up, and is in the fresh air.

3. Walking, Exercise, Physio (Physical) Therapy

It took me quite a while before my body was strong enough to even think about doing physiotherapy. It was not until I had SIBO, Candida, and pancreatic replacement therapy under control, and had been able to resolve many of the symptoms caused by nutrient deficiencies that I had the energy for one short session every two or three weeks. It would take days of recovery, which is a classic CFS symptom called post exertion malaise. It is ironic that exercise helps in reducing unhealthy mitochondria and increasing healthy volumes, as initially there is little energy (generated by mitochondria) available for any exercise. I had to ease into to it in order to slowly get muscles and joints to function again without injuring something due to long term non-use.

Very slowly I was able to build tolerance, and able to do small weights, some pushups and simple exercises. A little side note in terms of the immediate pancreatic impact, a few minutes of some simple exercises with dumbbells now easily drops my blood glucose level by twenty to thirty points. This in turn requires less insulin production by the pancreas.

Walking is always something to try, even during some of the worst moments, and even if it is only to street's edge, or the end of the block and back. Movement and exercise help with healing, neurotransmitter production, cleaning up of toxins and dysfunctional cells, improving mitochondrial function and blood circulation, to name a few. If you can handle it, try some yoga type movements and stretching, walk or move in a mineral water pool, or walk ankle deep in water at the lake's or ocean's edge. When you get a little stronger, try a little bike ride, or a few minutes of swimming. When you do start to be able to do a bit more cardio work, make sure to keep your heart rate (in beats per minute) in a healthy zone, on average not higher than 180 minus your age. Do what you can, but pace yourself

4. Mineral Baths

In Germany there is a concept of the healing power of water called Kneipp. It is named after Sebastian Kneipp who healed himself from, at the time incurable, tuberculosis through mineral bath therapy. He mentioned "spend a little bit of time now for your health, or a lot of time later with your illness." There are many salt (non-chlorinated!), mineral hot springs around the world known for its healing powers. Something so ancient, simple, and yet so powerful and relaxing can help heal in multiple ways:

• It allows essential minerals to soak in through your skin.

• It relaxes the mind and thus lowers the amount of nutrients needed on stress hormones and its negative impacts.

• It grounds you to the earth, reducing oxidative stress and inflammation.

It is also one of the reasons why surfing is so healthy. You get exposed to essential minerals from the ocean, grounding to the earth, full body exercise, fresh air, infra-red rays from the sun for mitochondrial health, ultraviolet B rays for vitamin D production, and just the sheer joy of it. But, until you are strong enough to go surfing again, just walking bare feet in the sea water is already helpful.

If you are not close to a mineral spring or the ocean, you can buy magnesium bath salt like Epsom, put 500 grams (just over a pound) in a warm bath, and soak for 20-30 minutes. Until I was strong enough to walk outside again, this was one of the few amazingly calming, pain reducing, and healing elements I did multiple times per week. Not to mention that it helps with magnesium deficiencies.

5. Sleep Hygiene

Get as much sleep as your body tells you to, as this is healing time. For many months after the bedridden phase, I would need to sleep all afternoon. This would provide me with a couple of hours per day of function, and it would help lower the pain. For a long time, my best time of the day was when I was unconscious. My body was essentially telling me in no uncertain terms that I needed to rest in order to heal. Nowadays, I still regularly have to take a short nap in the afternoon, which I combine with meditation. But, I let my body tell me when it is needed. In some cultures an afternoon siesta is perfectly acceptable.

Beside sleep quantity, quality is important. Another simple yet effective action you can take, if not done already, is to make the environment in which you sleep as optimal as possible. Use the best mattress you can afford, since you spend so much time on it per day. Get a pillow for in between your knees if you are side sleeper, in order to improve your spine position. Temperature control is important, so that you can make it cooler and allow fresh air in. Do not use any blue light devices an hour or so before going to sleep. For reading, do not use any LED, neon or halogen lights in the bedroom, but instead use old fashioned incandescent bulbs that have a natural spectrum of light. Remove, or turn off completely, any electronic devices during sleeping time. Reduce light pollution by making sure that all windows are covered to make it really dark, or use an eye mask. There should not be any LED or other lights shining in the room no matter how bright, as it can impact your circadian rhythm. Reduce the EMF field where you sleep, as this can impact your mitochondria. I do not have an alarm clock or a TV in the bedroom, and I turn off the electricity completely at the breaker panel for the whole bedroom before going to sleep. There are timers available to automate this if desired.

6. Pacing

There is an amazing book listed in the Appendix about Chronic Fatigue Syndrome, which mentions pacing yourself as a key element to heal. Do not do too much too quickly. Know when your body is sending you the message that you do not have energy for an activity. If you mentally push through, which is easy to do, you will pay the price. This is something I still need to be reminded of frequently, as it is so easy to overdo things when you feel even a glimmer of lower malaise and pain, or a slight increase in energy. So many times I jumped on doing what would be considered standard stuff for anyone healthy, like getting a haircut, or buying some groceries, when I was not quite ready for it. Such a simple activity could easily set me back a week or two. Who knew that getting a haircut could cause you to be bedridden for a few days!

Again, these are all classic ME/CFS symptoms, when you just cannot produce the level of ATP to function normally. You will learn to listen to your body over time to see how far you can push activities. It can be as simple as your eyesight getting a bit blurry, or a little muscle tremor, or it is suddenly a bit harder to understand what you are hearing or reading, etc. But until you stop the bleeding, so to speak, by reducing the burdens to the body, replenishing nutrient deficiencies and start healing, you will not have energy for anything but the healing process. It goes in cycles, and improvements can be very slow initially. Pacing yourself, being patient and aware of these cycles and setbacks is vital.

7. Grounding or Earthing

An activity as old as mankind, yet somehow little known in mainstream, often dismissed or deemed controversial. This is simply the healing impact of your body making contact with the earth. Walking barefoot, wading in the ocean, soaking in a mineral spring, even taking a shower will electrically connect you with the earth. We have all kinds of electrical currents flowing through our bodies. The simplest example is the small electrical impulses that keep our hearts ticking. Our bodies will naturally produce reactive oxygen species (ROS) either through mitochondrial ATP energy production, detoxification of environmental pollutants, or immune system functions. A subset of ROS are the highly reactive molecules known as free radicals, which are those with unpaired electrons. This is all normal biochemistry. Your body will strive for a tightly controlled homeostasis, where antioxidants balance the free radicals.

Earthing provides unpaired electrons from the earth's surface to flow into our bodies, serving as another "antioxidant" by pairing with unpaired electrons. Studies have shown that earthing can help with healing wounds, and can indirectly be anti-inflammatory. It basically helps reduce oxidative stress. If you have ever dipped your feet into the salt sea after feeling particularly stressed, you can almost feel the immediate relief. Placebo? Who cares, in this case.

8. Meditation, Visualization, Imagery Healing, Praying, Yoga, Mindfulness, De-Stressing

Whatever name you want to give it, or whichever technique you prefer to use, any method that helps you relax can lower stress levels and brings calmness to your mind and body. This can help with the healing process. There are a few books I added in the Appendix that have helped me in this area. Since stress level and mindset are powerful participants and influencers on healing, both consciously and subconsciously, they are important to look at. I needed to find coping tools to be able to better handle the negative changes in my life, the constant pain, malaise and subsequent depression. To be able to separate the illness itself from how you react to that illness is important in healing, the latter over which you have some control through meditation, visualization, imagery healing or yoga.

There are many forms of yoga, but for me it was the deep relaxation breathing exercises and meditation that really were the ones to help with lowering pain and malaise. At no time during my healing was I well enough, nor interested in the hot box group exercise sessions that have become so popular these days. There is a guided meditation app from Headspace that is a good place to start. I would often combine a guided meditation session with a hot Epsom salt mineral bath. Walking meditation in your garden or out in nature is also calming.

Visualization and imagery healing are another form of meditation, where you use imagery to bridge the gap between conscious and subconscious thoughts. This brings your mind into a relaxed state in order to help bring insights and positive healing thoughts into the process. I would often fall asleep during the meditation or visualization sessions, which just proves to me how relaxing the activity is.

Stress

Stress and the feeling of constantly being in fight or flight mode requires a lot of nutrients, which are in short supply for those with pancreas damage like EPI. It is a useful core survival mechanism to stop any unnecessary processes not immediately required for survival, and pump hormones such as adrenaline into the blood for extra awareness, speed and strength in order to avoid a life-threatening situation. When you are stressed you hinder your healing processes by using up nutrients needed elsewhere. Secondly, your body is put in a state which puts healing on pause, as it is a much lower priority to fight or flight.

These days your mind is put into a constant level of stress due to modern day pressures. Beside the usual daily stresses, a relatively new one is the information overload stress. Social media notifications, pushed news feeds, automatic updates to your phone with new postings, new messages, new emails, new text messages, new news articles, stock tickers, new likes, etc. are all part of these information feedback loops that constantly trigger hormones like dopamine and adrenaline in your body. Social media is physically addictive. Try to turn them all off for large blocks of time. Instead, set aside a very specific short time period when, if you even have the energy, you check and reply to information demands. I completely unplugged from all social media and automated data pushes to conserve precious energy.

The released stress hormones impact sleep quality, healing processes, compromise your immune system, and increase systemic inflammation.

<u>Additional Health Stress</u>

Here are a few examples of additional daily stresses that come into play when you are not healthy. Healthcare, unemployment or disability insurances are often linked to your job. Lose your job and you lose your healthcare insurance for the family. Medical and medicine bills are very expensive. Over $600 out-of-pocket for the first month of pancreatic enzymes? Check. An ambulance trip that is not "in network" of the insurance? That ten-minute trip to the emergency room just cost $2,500 out-of-pocket. An emergency room doctor who does not accept your insurance, even when you went to the "in-network" hospital, with subsequent massive bills? Check. $9,000 MRI? Check. $1,200 for a thirty minute doctor's visit in the hospital? Check. 200$ extra "facility fee" for that same doctor's visit just because the doctor had his office inside the hospital? Check. An emergency doctor's ordered hospital stay that the insurance declines to pay for? Check. Spending countless hours battling insurance companies because they suddenly decide that the blood tests ordered by the doctor are "experimental" or not a "medical necessity" in their opinion, causing you to have to pay the insanely inflated, (sometimes ten-fold) non-discounted list price of the laboratory? Check.

Of course, all of these absurd prices and the insurance small print are only known to you after the fact, when you open the medical bill and get another stress shock to the system!

De-stress

The reason I bring up these examples is that consciously and subconsciously this adds an additional burden to the body at a time when you are trying to heal. Really do not underestimate the negative impact of stress and the importance of using tools such as meditation to lower the stress level. Meditation, yoga, visualization, or de-stressing in any of the various forms can help the healing process.

Some potential benefits are that it can:

- Relax blood vessels and improve blood circulation.
- Improve lymphatic system circulation to support the immune system, cellular debris removal, and transport of white blood cells.
- Lower stress and thus related hormone production.
- Improve mood and lower depression.
- Improve immune system and lower inflammation.
- Lower pain.
- Lower blood pressure and heart rate.

Simple Meditation Example

Meditation and visualization have really helped me with handling pain and improving my mood. I still try to do one or two, roughly twenty minute, sessions per day. During the meditation I usually follow these steps, but the process will be different and personal for everyone.

Step 1. Get comfortable. I usually lie on my back with a blanket over me, an eye cover to block all light, and a pillow under my head. If it is noisy I put in ear plugs as well.

Step 2. Take a few deep, slow, belly breaths; in through the nose and out through the mouth. I visualize breathing in healing energy and spreading it across different parts of my body. When breathing out I try to let go of tension, stress, thoughts and pain, and just focus on breathing in and out.

Step 3. Focus slowly on each area of the body to relax it, starting at the toes and feet, and moving slowly up each muscle group. You might be surprised how many small muscles are tense without realizing it, including your jaw and face muscles. After a while my hands start to warm up indicating blood vessels are relaxing, and there is more blood circulation.

Step 4. Starting at the top of my head I mentally flow down my body and focus on areas that are particularly painful or unhealthy. I visualize flowing healing energy and warmth (some people like imagining a light, or cool stream instead) to those areas. I try to visualize the anatomy and focus on specific organs or pain areas.

Step 5. I imagine myself walking through a path in the forest towards a peaceful spot. For me this is always a serene place in nature with spectacular views, no people, no noise, and no pollution. Either it is a scene I remember from my travels (New Zealand is a fav), or an imagination of where I would like to be, like a sunny deserted beach. Find your "happy" place. If thoughts start to interrupt, I will focus back on just breathing in and out.

Step 6. When I have settled in, I imagine how I would like to be in the future. I visualize doing an activity that I love, and feeling healthy enough to be able to perform it. One example for me involves blasting over an open ocean on a windsurfer.

Step 7. By this time I often fall asleep. Sleeping is healing!

There is really no wrong way to meditate, as long as you try to relax. When your body no longer feels it is in fight or flight mode it can start focusing more attention, energy and resources to healing. Blood vessels and the lymphatic system relax, which improves the circulation of nutrients and immune system cells, and helps clean up cellular garbage.

9. Light

Certain light frequencies are healing to mitochondria, important in ATP energy production, affect mood and sleep, and help vitamin D production to name a few benefits.

Sunlight is of course best. It provides the healing effect of infra-red light on the mitochondria. It also provides ultraviolet B light to help the body produce vitamin D, potentially lowering cholesterol in the process as it used as a raw material. These days, the little time spent outdoors, and then often with sun blocking cream, is a big influence on widespread vitamin D insufficiency. A healthy sunlight amount is around 15-20 minutes of full body exposure per day. You might have heard of light therapy as a way to help with seasonal affective disorder (SAD), or excessive exposure to artificial light. Growing up in the Northern hemisphere, it was not uncommon to get some light therapy in the midst of winter.

Since these days we spend many hours of the day inside, the type of lights you use in the house is very important. Do not use LED, neon, or fluorescent lights in the areas where you live or sleep. LED is a digital light which flickers constantly at a very high frequency, produces high levels of blue light and has little of the healing frequencies. Stick with old-school incandescent light bulbs, as they have a more complete light spectrum, close to daylight, and contain more of the healing light spectrum. Sadly, this forced move to low power consumption lights has ignored the direct health impact. Not to mention that most of those energy efficient lamps are considered toxic waste.

On a side note, also try to lower the blue light impact of your computer screens, tablets, and phone, as it increases reactive oxygen species (ROS) and thus can increase oxidative stress. Many electronic items now have a setting for this.

10. Electro-Magnetic Fields (EMF)

Getting the electro-magnetic radiation exposure under control, as much as is realistic, can help stem another burden to your mitochondria, and in turn help the healing process. This is another area that is not well-known in mainstream medicine and often ridiculed, even though there are many studies showing the negative impact of EMF on the body. It can cause mitochondrial or DNA damage, and even cancer, with strong and long enough exposure.

Of course you are bombarded all day by EMF that you cannot avoid, so again the idea here is that every little bit helps in reducing the burden to your body in order to help it get back to homeostasis. There are a few easy actions that you can do, since many sources we have no control over. Here are a few examples:

Lower Micro Wave Exposure

• Do not stand within two meters of the microwave oven when it is running.

• Put your phone in airplane mode, or off, when it is close to your body or in your pocket. There are even some EMF phone guards available these days.

• Turn off the bluetooth radio on your phone, tablet or computer when not using it.

• Turn off the Wi-Fi radio on your phone, tablet or computer when not using it.

• Use a wired headset when making a call.

• Do not hold the phone close to your body or in your hand when making a call, or when any of the radio transmitters are on, such as bluetooth, Wi-Fi or cellular. Do not keep your phone close to your bed, or turn it off completely when sleeping.

• Get rid of any DECT style wireless home phones, as they are like having a microwave oven running all day long, with a huge range of radiation. Replace it with an old fashioned wired one instead.

• Use wired internet connections for your laptop or computer instead of Wi-Fi whenever possible.

• Use a separate wired, instead of wireless, keyboard and mouse, so that you put some distance between the laptop and your body.

• Use EMF shielding for utility smart meters and Wi-Fi routers, if they are close to where you sleep or work.

Lower Electrical Field Exposure

• Consider having your house checked for unhealthy EMF levels. You can either use a simple EMF meter, or have a professional check your house. When you live extremely close to, for example, electrical substations, or high voltage lines this might be worth it. But, most EMF actually comes from within your house, for example, from electricity lines if not in conduits, or electronics.

• Consider turning off the electricity breaker in your bedroom before going to sleep, or have them on a timer. In many cities electrical wiring does not have to be in metal conduits, which means you can measure the EMF field from the wires at least 2-3 meters (~6.5-10 feet) away from the wall. My bedroom had been tested with unhealthy EMF levels showing from the head of the bed, where electrical wiring was in the wall, all the way to the foot of the bed. I notice a sense of calmness with the electricity turned off in the bedroom, and I sleep better.

• Do not have your laptop directly on your lap, but instead use a small laptop table, or an EMF shield.

• Look into EMF shields for electronic components with a large field, or those that are close to your body during work or sleep. For example, utility smart meters, wireless routers, wireless chargers, wall warts, fans, regulators, amplifiers, fridges, light ballasts, etc.

• When using your laptop and you have the power plugged in to charge, the EMF field is much larger. Try to use battery power as much as possible.

• Do not have appliances (e.g. a fridge) close to where you spend much of your time, for example, where you sleep or work.

• Do not use LED, neon or fluorescent lights in the areas where you live or sleep, as they not only flicker at high speeds, cause high pitched noise, but can also throw a large EMF field.

The Future

My hope in writing this book was to provide you with some insights, useful information, and practical steps to consider. Perhaps highlight some new avenues to pursue in your quest for better health, with a glimmer of hope that things can get better. By following the steps I shared here I was able to go from death's door to a functioning human being again, even with just a sliver of the pancreas left. Hopefully, these steps will help you (or your patients) improve as well.

You will probably go through all the usual mental stages of trauma during this process. The acceptance portion was tough for me, but it is what stubbornly kept me going to find solutions. I could not accept that the remainder of my life would have devolved into being a prisoner of my bed or couch, dependent on my wife for everything, in order to just survive in pain and malaise. But, it will not be easy and will require patience and determination, as you will likely hit roadblocks and setbacks along the way. Often during the healing period it will feel like you are on a rollercoaster, where one minute you are starting to feel better, and the next you get slammed again. But slowly, the up periods will become longer than the down periods.

Throughout the healing process, always keep a few goals in mind. My goals are to go on vacation with my wife again, to be able to stand on a windsurfer and blast through white caps during forty km/h winds, or stand on my motorbike riding through off-road passages. Remind yourself of why you want to get better. It would be amazing if I can prove my doctors wrong, and show that acinar cell regeneration is a possibility, even when over ninety percent of them have been atrophied away. However, that is more of a fantasy until perhaps medical technology provides a new solution in the future. For those of you in the pre-EPI phase, with more acinar cells left, this might very well be something to strive for!

Depending on how hard your pancreas was hit, you will have to be very careful with your body and what you consume for the rest of your life, in order not to regress. Please do not get complacent just because you are feeling better.

Of course, microbiome health and nutrient deficiencies will still have to be monitored. Pancreatic enzymes will be required with every meal, and supplementation will still be important, albeit far less than during the healing period. Continue to pay close attention to what you eat and drink, especially when eating out, as the microbiome can deteriorate rapidly. Try to always minimize the daily bodily insults of excess sugar, bad tap water, herbicides, pesticides, bad air, chemicals and plastic exposure. Be kind to your pancreas and your body.

When you have gone through the process of healing, you will be more in tune with your body. You will be able to recognize more quickly when you have overdone it, or digested something unhealthy and inflammatory. Listen to your body, as it really tries to give you hints! Your body is an amazing piece of machinery that constantly strives hard for homeostasis; a healthy equilibrium.

Please continue with your determination to improve your health. I wish you all the best and strength in your journey!!!

APPENDIX

References

Through the years of struggling to find answers about my health, and searching for any information that could possibly help in healing, I came across many books, articles, blogs, and research documents. Some days I could barely read a sentence, but Dr. Google, PubMed and the NCBI became my friends. I am thankful to all who shared their information and research.

Below I mention a few from which I learnt a lot, and could be worth looking at if you want to dig deeper. They are in no particular order.

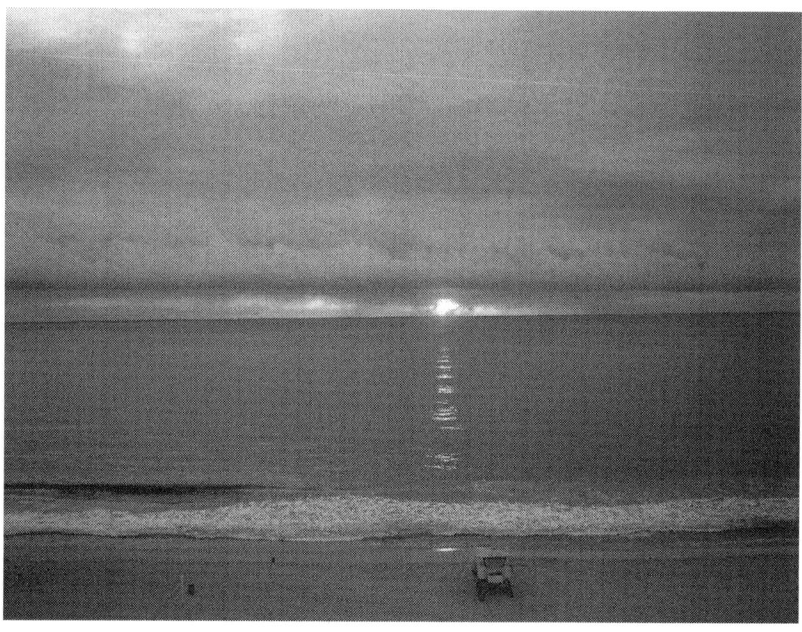

1. Medical Research

An amazing source of research reports, studies and medical information. Over the years there are too many studies and reports I have read on these biomedical websites to mention. I am grateful to all the researchers who shared their studies.

- **National Center for Biotechnology Information**

https://www.ncbi.nlm.nih.gov/

- **US National Library of Medicine**

https://www.nlm.nih.gov/

- **PubMed**

https://www.ncbi.nlm.nih.gov/pubmed/

- **National Institutes of Health**

https://www.nih.gov/

2. Food and Diet

Mark Sisson. A great source of paleo and primal lifestyle, nutrition and health information are Mark Sisson's websites, books and podcasts. Podcasts can be downloaded to your phone, containing great interviews, with a wide variety of guests, from doctors who have seen the light, to nutrition specialists.

- The New Primal Blueprint
- The Keto Reset Diet

https://www.marksdailyapple.com/

http://blog.primalblueprint.com/

https://www.marksdailyapple.com/primal-blueprint-101/

https://www.marksdailyapple.com/healthy-oils/

Dr. William Davis. An eye opening book on the dangers of modern wheat on the body:

- Wheat Belly

http://www.wheatbellyblog.com/

Dr. Jamie Koufman and **Dr. Jordan Stern.** When I could barely tolerate any food with many acid reflux issues, this book helped:

- Dropping Acid – The Reflux Diet Cookbook and Cure

Dr. Stephen T. Sinatra. Great explanation by a cardiologist of the link between heart issues, CFS, nutrition, and supplementation, in particular CoQ10:

- The Sinatra Solution: Metabolic Cardiology

Dr. William G. Crook. A book on an anti-yeast diet:

- The Yeast Connection

Dr. Catherine Shanahan. A book on nutrition and the dangers of certain foods:

- Deep Nutrition: Why Your Genes Need Traditional Food

Dr. David Servan-Schreiber M.D. PhD. An MD who used food, supplements and lifestyle changes to survive many extra years after brain cancer diagnosis:

- Anticancer: A New Way of Life

• **AGE foods info**. Advanced Glycation End Products in Foods and a Practical Guide to Their Reduction in the Diet by Dr. Jaime Uribarri et al.:

https://www.ncbi.nlm.nih.gov/pmc/articles/PMC3704564/

• **Principles of Human Nutrition**: Johns Hopkins Bloomberg School of Public Health:

http://ocw.jhsph.edu/courses/humannutrition/lectureNotes.cfm

https://global.oup.com/uk/orc/biosciences/molbiol/snape_biochemistry5e/student/weblinks/

• **An example of sugar impact.** Sugar Industry and Coronary Heart Disease Research. A Historical Analysis of Internal Industry Documents. A Historical Analysis of Internal Industry Documents by Cristin E. Kearns et al.:

https://www.ncbi.nlm.nih.gov/pmc/articles/PMC5099084/

3. Water

• **Environmental Working Group (EWG).** Find tap water quality in the USA based on zip code:

https://www.ewg.org/tapwater/

• **Fluoride health impact.** Information on the negative health impacts of fluoride:

https://www.epa.gov/sites/production/files/documents/tsca_21_petition_hfsa_2013-04-22.pdf

http://fluoridealert.org

• **Dangers of Demineralized Water.** World Health Organization study on demineralized water impact on the body:

https://www.who.int/water_sanitation_health/dwq/nutrientschap12.pdf

• **Minerals in Drinking Water.** World Health Organization study on essential minerals in water and their health impact:

https://www.who.int/water_sanitation_health/dwq/nutrientsindw.pdf

• **EPA National Primary Drinking Water Regulations:**

https://www.epa.gov/ground-water-and-drinking-water/national-primary-drinking-water-regulations

4. Toxins

• **Environmental Working Group (EWG).** An organization sharing a wealth of information and research studies on the impacts on health from, e.g., herbicides, chemicals, etc.:

https://www.ewg.org/key-issues/toxics/pesticides

• **World Health Organization International Agency for Research on Cancer.** Information on a variety of pesticides, herbicides, and chemicals:

https://www.iarc.fr/

https://monographs.iarc.fr/wp-content/uploads/2018/08/14-002.pdf

Plastics, BPA, phthalates, polystyrene, per- and poly-fluorinated chemicals (PFC)

• **Environmental Working Group**

https://www.ewg.org/research/many-fast-food-wrappers-still-coated-pfcs-kin-carcinogenic-teflon-chemical https://www.ewg.org/key-issues/consumer-products/food-containers

• **Safer Chemicals, Healthy Families**

https://saferchemicals.org/get-the-facts/

https://saferchemicals.org/2014/05/26/styrene-and-styrofoam-101-2/

• **Toxic-Free Future**

https://toxicfreefuture.org/

Glyphosate herbicide

Starting points from where you can find additional research links:

• California Proposition 65 listing

https://oehha.ca.gov/proposition-65/crnr/glyphosate-listed-effective-july-7-2017-known-state-california-cause-cancer

• World Health Organization – International Agency for Research on Cancer:

https://monographs.iarc.fr/wp-content/uploads/2018/06/mono112-10.pdf

• Glyphosate patents: Chelating Agent, U.S. patent number 3160632 A. Herbicide, U.S. patent number 3455675 A. Anti-microbial, U.S. patent number 20040077608 A1. Biocide, U.S. patent number 7771736 B2. Details and patent office links can be found here:

http://www.gmofreepartners.com/wp-content/uploads/2015/04/glyphosate-patents.pdf

https://patents.google.com/

• Glyphosate, pathways to modern diseases: celiac, sprue and gluten intolerance by Anthony Samsel and Stephanie Seneff. They are often dismissed as controversial, so do your own reading and follow the trail of research they have analyzed.

https://www.ncbi.nlm.nih.gov/pubmed/24678255

https://www.drperlmutter.com/empowering-neurologist-dr-stephanie-seneff/

https://drpompa.com/additional-resources/health-tips/the-dangers-of-glyphosate-an-interview-with-dr-stephanie-seneff

Atrazine pesticide

• Agency for Toxic Substances & Disease Registry:

https://www.atsdr.cdc.gov/phs/phs.asp?id=336&tid=59

• World Health Organization International Agency for Research on Cancer:

https://monographs.iarc.fr/wp-content/uploads/2018/06/TR42-19.pdf

https://www.iarc.fr/

5. Chronic Fatigue Syndrome (ME/CFS)

Dr. Sarah Myhill. A great ME/CFS book I encountered in describing and explaining the many symptoms, causes, tests as well as a lot of information on beneficial supplements:

• Diagnosis and Treatment of Chronic Fatigue Syndrome and Myalgic Encephalitis: It's Mitochondria, Not Hypochondria

• Chronic fatigue syndrome and mitochondrial dysfunction http://www.ijcem.com/files/IJCEM812001.pdf

http://www.drmyhill.co.uk/wiki/CFS_-_The_Central_Cause:_Mitochondrial_Failure

• **The Mitochondrial Medicine Society.** Information on mitochondrial dysfunctions:

http://www.mitosoc.org/

• A Modern Approach to the Treatment of Mitochondrial Disease by Sumit Parikh, MD, Russell Saneto, DO, PhD and The Mitochondrial Medicine Society:

https://www.ncbi.nlm.nih.gov/pmc/articles/PMC3561461/

• Great websites for those suffering with ME/CFS, with people sharing their stories and knowledge:

http://phoenixrising.me/

https://www.healthrising.org/

https://www.meaction.net/

6. Exocrine Pancreatic Insufficiency (EPI)

• **EPI.** Great explanation of EPI by Dr. Samer Al-Kaade:

https://emedicine.medscape.com/article/2121028-overview#a7

• Practical guide to exocrine pancreatic insufficiency – Breaking the myths by M.R. Struyvenberg, C. R. Martin, S.D. Freedman

https://www.ncbi.nlm.nih.gov/pmc/articles/PMC5301368/

Creon. The pancreatic enzyme manufacturer who makes Creon has a good introductory website on EPI and pancrelipase:

https://www.creon.com/how-creon-works

• **EPI Testing.** Pancreatic function testing: Here to stay for the 21st century by John G Lieb II and Peter V Draganov: https://www.ncbi.nlm.nih.gov/pmc/articles/PMC2712845/

• **Pancreatic enzyme replacement therapy** for pancreatic exocrine insufficiency in the 21st century Tony Trang, Johanna Chan, and David Y Graham: https://www.ncbi.nlm.nih.gov/pmc/articles/PMC4155341/

The link between exocrine and endocrine pancreas damage. Here are a few examples, but if you search PubMed you will find many similar studies:

• Exocrine Pancreatic Insufficiency in Diabetes Mellitus: A Complication of Diabetic Neuropathy or a Different Type of Diabetes?:

https://www.ncbi.nlm.nih.gov/pmc/articles/PMC3148449/#B21

• Interactions between the endocrine and exocrine pancreas and their clinical relevance by Czakó L et al.:

https://www.ncbi.nlm.nih.gov/pubmed/19454837

• World Journal of Gastroenterology. Relationship between the exocrine and endocrine pancreas after acute pancreatitis by Stephanie L. M. Das et al.:

https://www.wjgnet.com/1007-9327/full/v20/i45/17196.htm

• Journal of the Pancreas (http://www.joplink.net/) had an international workshop quite a while ago, but there are many linked research reports here that can be of interest:

http://www.joplink.net/prev/200807/07.html

7. Microbiome

Microbiome importance. PubMed and NCBI have a wealth of information available on the subject.

• The gut microbiome in health and in disease by Andrew B. Shreiner, John Y. Kao, and Vincent B. Young:

https://www.ncbi.nlm.nih.gov/pmc/articles/PMC4290017/

• A SIBO and EPI link example. Small intestinal bacterial overgrowth syndrome by Bures J. et al.:

https://www.ncbi.nlm.nih.gov/pubmed/20572300

8. Nutrition, Supplements, Organic Acid Tests, Biochemistry

Biochemistry textbook with a wealth of information on metabolic pathways, nutrient cofactors, health and sickness as a function of biochemistry:

• Harper's Illustrated Biochemistry by Victor W. Rodwell and David Bender

Organic Acid Test Interpretations and Guides. A wealth of information is available for the interpretation of organic acid nutritional testing, the citric acid cycle and metabolic pathways. When you complete a nutrition organic acid lab test, the results report also provides some information. But, sometimes you might want to dig a little deeper.

• **Great Plains Laboratory**

https://www.greatplainslaboratory.com/oat-book/

• **Genova Diagnostics** (Also Metametrix) has great interpretive guides on subjects from fatty acids, citric acid cycle, amino acids, toxins, to oxidative stress and more. The ION-IG.pdf has a great chart explaining the citric acid cycle on the last page:

https://www.gdx.net/core/interpretive-guides/Fatty-Acids-IG.pdf

https://www.gdx.net/core/interpretive-guides/ION-IG.pdf

https://www.gdx.net/core/interpretive-guides/Toxic-Effects-CORE-Interp-Guide.pdf

https://www.gdx.net/core/interpretive-guides/Oxidative-Stress-Interp-Guide.pdf

• **ARL** functional pathology Urinary Organic Acids Guide:

http://www.peirsoncenter.com/uploads/6/0/5/5/6055321/1216.urinary_organic_acids.pdf

• **Functional Diagnostic Medicine Training Program** Insider's Guide Interpretation and Treatment: Organic Acid – Energy and Oxidative Markers and Treatment by Ron Grisanti, D.C. and Dicken Weatherby, N.D.:

http://www.functionalmedicine.net/pdf/Insider%27s%20Guide_37.pdf

• **Amino Acid and Protein Requirements.** World Health Organization - Protein and amino acid requirements in human nutrition report of a joint FAO/WHO/UNU expert consultation:

http://apps.who.int/iris/handle/10665/43411

• **Micronutrients**: Linus Pauling Institute Micronutrient Information Center is a great source of nutrient information:

https://lpi.oregonstate.edu/mic

https://lpi.oregonstate.edu/publications/micronutrients-health

https://lpi.oregonstate.edu/mic/vitamins

https://lpi.oregonstate.edu/mic/minerals

https://lpi.oregonstate.edu/mic/other-nutrients/essential-fatty-acids

https://lpi.oregonstate.edu/mic/other-nutrients/choline

• **Micronutrients**: Dr. Jacob Teitelbaum has good information regarding CFS and nutrition:

http://www.vitality101.com/nutrition-overview/herbals-vitamins-and-minerals

• **Omega-6 Imbalance.** Health Implications of High Dietary omega-6 Polyunsaturated Fatty Acids by E. Patterson and company:

https://www.ncbi.nlm.nih.gov/pmc/articles/PMC3335257/

• **L-Serine** Supplementation Attenuates Alcoholic Fatty Liver by Enhancing Homocysteine Metabolism in Mice and Rats by Woo-Cheol Sim and company. The Journal of Nutrition, Volume 145, Issue 2, 1 February 2015, Pages 260–267:

https://academic.oup.com/jn/article/145/2/260/4644338

• **Other nutrition sites:**

https://academic.oup.com/jn

https://nutritionreview.org

https://www.lifeextension.com has a magazine with interesting articles. They do sell supplements, but the information is free.

https://deannaminich.com/vitamin-and-mineral-interactions-the-complex-relationship-of-essential-nutrients/

9. Functional or Integrative Medicine

Some doctors who understand the importance of food and supplements, and share great info in their books and websites. As with anything you read these days, check credentials, wonder about monetary motivations, be critical, and hold on to your common sense. Some have written things that are controversial, and others have a monetary benefit from anything they advertise and sell on their websites. I have just used it to gather information that could possibly benefit me and have ignored any products that they might sell. Luckily there are more integrative medicine practices in some of the top medical institutions, with medical doctors specializing in it, albeit it with long waiting lists. But, do not just dismiss information if it is not coming from an M.D.

- Dr. Hyman:
https://drhyman.com/

- Dr. Perlmutter:
https://www.drperlmutter.com/

- Dr. Charles Moss:
http://mosscenterforintegrativemedicine.com/

- Dr. Weil:
https://www.drweil.com/

- Dr. Stephen Sinatra:
https://www.drsinatra.com/about-dr-sinatra

- Dr. Gordon Saxe:
https://extension.ucsd.edu/about-extension/gordon-saxe

- Josh Axe:
https://draxe.com/

- Chris Kresser:
https://chriskresser.com/

10. Other Healing Elements

• **Meditation.** Rituals of Healing: Using Imagery for Health and Wellness by Jeanne Achterberg, PhD and Barbara Dossey, PhD.

• **Meditation.** Guided Imagery for Self-Healing by Dr. Martin L.Rossman

• **EMF.** Electro Magnetic Field radiation and its health impact information:

https://en.geovital.com/

• PubMed has studies on the EMF impact on mitochondria, for example:

https://www.ncbi.nlm.nih.gov/pubmed/?term=mitochondria+EMF

• **Intelligent Scale.** Bio-electrical impedance analysis (BIA) technology:

https://www.tanita.com/en/understanding-your-measurements/

• **Grounding.** The effects of grounding (earthing) on inflammation, the immune response, wound healing, and prevention and treatment of chronic inflammatory and autoimmune diseases by James L Oschman, Gaétan Chevalier, and Richard Brown:

https://www.ncbi.nlm.nih.gov/pmc/articles/PMC4378297/

• **LED Lighting.** Effect of LED lighting on health examples:

https://articles.mercola.com/sites/articles/archive/2016/10/23/near-infrared-led-lighting.aspx

https://www.ncbi.nlm.nih.gov/pmc/articles/PMC3948029/

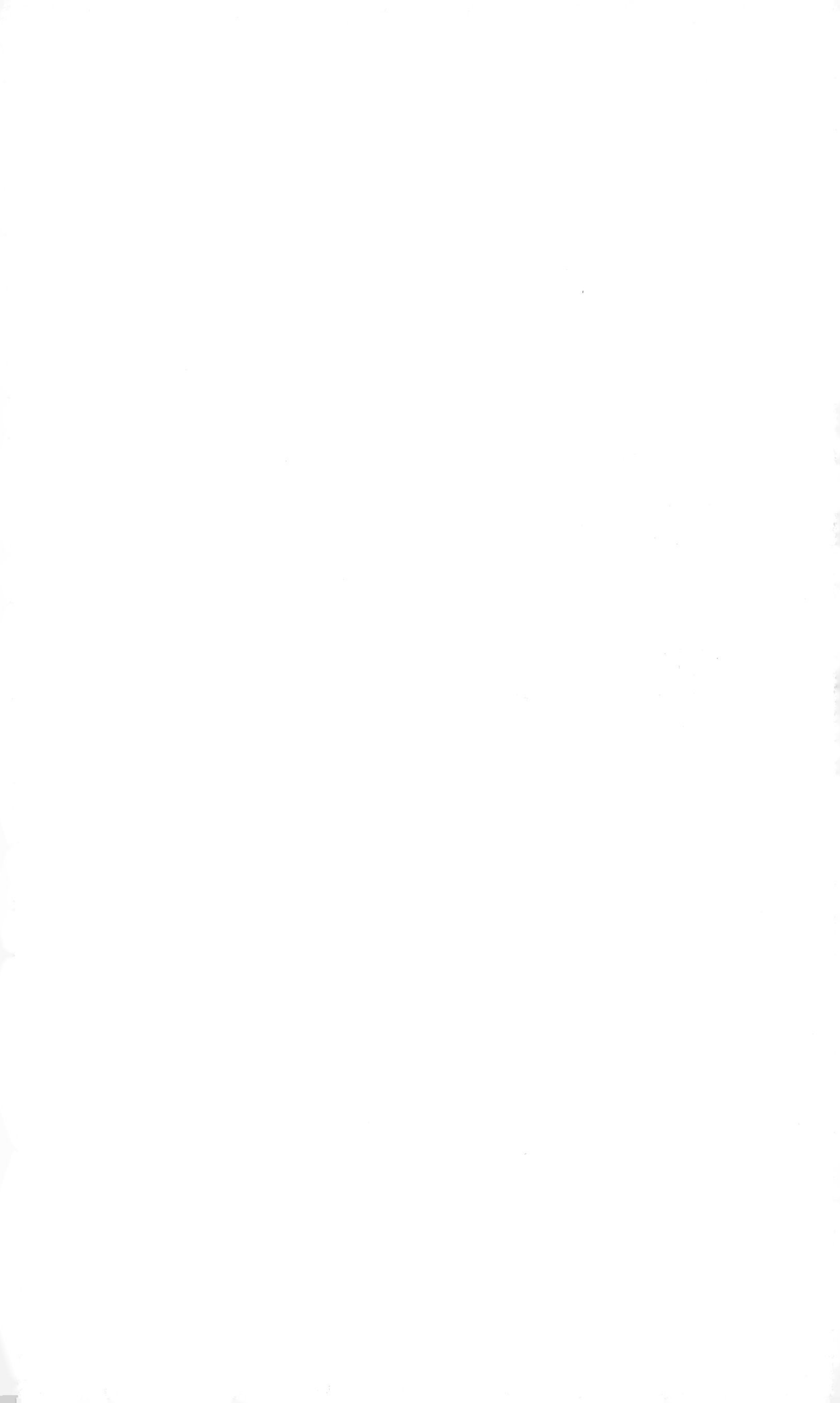

Made in United States
Orlando, FL
02 March 2023

30589213R00183